AGE STRONGER, LIVE LONGER

A Practical Guide to Optimal Health and Longevity

By Dr. Mani Kukreja

Age Stronger, Live Longer:
A Practical Guide to Optimal Health and Longevity

Copyright © Mani Kukreja (2025)

All rights reserved. No part of this publication may be reproduced, stored in a retrieval system, or transmitted, in any form or by any means, without the prior written permission of the publisher.

ISBN Paperback: 979-8-89576-101-4

Dr. Mani Kukreja holds an MBBS degree and a Master of Public Health (MPH) in Clinical Research. She is not currently practicing medicine. This book is intended to provide general wellness guidance and health optimization advice. It does not constitute medical advice, diagnosis, or treatment.

Table of Contents

Introduction 4

Chapter 1: What Ages Us? 8

Chapter 2: The Role of Age-Related Diseases 25

Chapter 3: Three Core Processes That Age Us 41

Chapter 4: The Hidden Impact of Environmental And Mental Stressors 48

Chapter 5: Lifestyle, Supplements, And Longevity Connection 60

Chapter 6: Optimal Diet - What, When, How to Eat 75

Chapter 7: Sleep Is the Key to Longevity 92

Chapter 8: Measure Yourself - If You Don't Measure, You Can't Manage 105

Chapter 9: Skin Health and Beauty – Unlocking the Radiance Within 117

Chapter 10: Movement, Strength, And Fitness – Foundation for Vitality 144

Conclusion: The Stronger Path Forward 154

References 156

Introduction

"It is not the years in your life that count, but the life in your years."
—Abraham Lincoln

I want to share a part of my life journey that is deeply personal, and profoundly relevant to many of us navigating stress, inflammation, and the complexities of our own health.

Let's dive in.

How we define "aging" is typically shaped by societal expectations of decline in parameters like appearance and function, metabolism, memory, fitness, immune function, and hormones. But aging does not have to mean decline.

While we are not immortal and will eventually die, how we live in the years we have is what matters. When we make the right choices, we can preserve vitality, and function long into life.

What many don't realize is that aging is not simply the passage of time—it's a complex biological process marked by the accumulation of oxidative stress and chronic inflammation. When these factors overwhelm the body, health begins to deteriorate. Think of it this way: A healthy body relies on balanced signaling molecules that keep inflammation in check. But when this balance is disrupted, inflammation damages essential cellular components like nucleic acids, proteins, and fatty acids. As a result of which our natural detoxification systems—the enzymes designed to cleanse our bodies, begin to falter under this pressure. It sets off a cycle of chronic inflammation that weakens our immune system and accelerates aging.

At age 52, I'm healthier, mentally sharper, and more physically fit than ever. I take pride in that not because of vanity, but because it reflects deliberate, consistent effort. And I've helped many others do the same.

Let me share both my professional/academic background and personal story.

Through over a decade of conducting clinical research on chronic diseases like cardiovascular disease, diabetes, and cancer, I uncovered two vital truths:

1. Our overall health declines rapidly as these diseases progress.
2. Targeted integrative interventions can often prevent, manage, or even reverse these conditions.

Personally, not too long ago, I faced a pivotal moment. At the height of my career, while juggling a demanding high-level role and the responsibilities of motherhood, I hit a wall. As a type-A personality, I thrived on achievement, but chronic stress took a toll on my immune system.

Instead of protecting me, my immune cells began attacking my own tissues, a condition called 'Autoimmune Disease.' As a result, I began experiencing fatigue, brain fog, and significant hair thinning—symptoms that I initially dismissed as stress. I later learned I was facing Hashimoto's thyroiditis, a condition where immune system targets the thyroid gland, resulting in fatigue and other hypothyroid symptoms.

Soon after, a shingles outbreak, a flare-up of the herpes virus, sent a louder signal that my immune system was under a serious strain. It was wake up call.

This experience taught me something profound: Our bodies speak to us in whispers long before they scream. If we ignore the subtle signs—fatigue, hair loss, brain fog—we may eventually face more significant, debilitating health challenges.

My healing journey has been about restoring and reestablishing balance, recognizing the deep connections between stress, inflammation, immunity and health. If my story resonates with you, I encourage you to listen to your body and recognize those early signs before they escalate into significant. Your body is always communicating.

This journey has revealed something powerful: When we address the root cause of disease and apply targeted lifestyle interventions, we don't just manage illness but we transform our health.

My Goals for You

We envision a future where our lifespan is balanced with an extended health span—where we not only live longer but also remain active and independent for as many of those years as possible. A future where age related ailments don't rob us of time with loved ones or our quality of life. This is what it truly means to age gracefully, "not just adding years to life, but life to years".

It all begins with understanding the "agers"— the key biological factors that influence how quickly or slowly we age. These include chronic inflammation, oxidative stress, hormone imbalances, and several other cellular processes I'll explore with you in the chapters ahead.

With the help of science backed tools and practical lifestyle strategies, we can intervene. These include sleep optimization, movement, personalized supplementation, photo modulation, heat and cold exposure, laser therapies, plasma-rich protein, hormone and peptide therapy, and red and infrared light exposure, and more. Together these interventions can supercharge our body's natural ability to heal, repair and rejuvenate.

Living longer is only truly meaningful if those added years are spent with a healthy body, a clear mind, vibrant energy, and strong immunity.

Life is *beautiful*. Live it *well*.

CHAPTER 1

What Ages Us?

While our age reflects how many years we've been alive, **aging** refers to how well our body has handled the journey throughout those years. That means AGING refers to both lifespan and quality of life combined. Some people age "better" than others or may even seem to not age at all despite decades having passed. Some people die in their 50s or 60s, while others live past 100. Some seem 20 years younger than others' biological age, while others appear decades older. These findings suggest that certain factors help people live and stay in better health for longer.

But what exactly is aging, and why do we age?

In this chapter, we'll start with a solid foundation on aging and what I consider the hallmarks of aging, or "**Agers**." Let's start with a few simple explanations, and then we'll take a more scientific look at what ages our bodies on a cellular level.

What Is Aging?

Aging is one of the most complex biological processes that exists, and defining it is no easy feat, even for the experts. According to *Aging: The Biology of Senescence,* "Aging is the time-related deterioration of the physiological functions necessary for survival and fertility." (Gilbert, 2000)

Aging is a process that affects almost all major organs and body systems. The rate at which aging affects the body will vary greatly from one person to the next. Moreover, how "well" we age is typically characterized by:

- Changes in appearance
- Reaction times
- Memory function
- Metabolism
- Fitness levels
- Sex drive
- Ability to see, hear, smell, etc.
- Decrease in organ function
- Weakened immune system
- Various hormonal changes

The truth is the "aging syndrome" takes root early on, in our mid-twenties, and operates invisibly for a long time (for most of us). The healthy levels we once had are now considered "reserves" and are starting to get depleted and are now dependent on interventions for replenishment.

By middle age, between our 30s and 40s, our cells are weak and shrinking because of drastic stem cell reduction, membranes become less permeable, muscle mass reduces, joints stiffen, thinning blood vessels impact our circulation and airway pathways, and our hormone levels also drastically decrease. These age-related symptoms happen at varying rates for different people, depending on how the different "agers" affect our bodies.

Why Do We Age?

The concept of aging has fascinated humans for centuries. There are a variety of interesting theories about the root cause of aging. Philosophers, scientists, and researchers have long debated the true causes of aging, resulting in many science-backed premises that generally fall into two major groups:

1. Many theories propose that aging is simply the result of a constant assault on our body's various cells, their proteins, and DNA. This assault on cells includes everything from environmental exposure and toxic byproducts to general inefficiencies in our body's natural repair system. The primary culprits are unstable atoms, ions, or molecules known as **free radicals**, which damage our cells and impair our repair mechanisms, accelerating the aging process. The damage (**free radicals**) accumulates like junk inside us throughout our lifespan, prompting some biological systems to fail. This, in turn, both causes and accelerates the aging process.

2. Some suggest that aging is predestined, based on and encoded in genes. They propose that these genes are somehow activated and cause a sequence of age-related changes and diseases. This happens on a fixed molecular clock that activates these sequences when we have served our purpose to humanity (reproduction). This "destiny" theory is rooted in the fact that we wear out our usefulness over time. However, we also know that this usefulness can vary

tremendously from person to person. There is no true evidence of this "genetic clock," and if there was, we all would be aging and dying at the same rate.

Aging is the mother of virtually **all diseases**, including most infectious diseases (Niccoli, 2012). So, if we can figure out how to improve our body's aging process, it's likely that we can also reduce our risk of chronic metabolic diseases, which are major "killers" listed below. More than two-thirds of all deaths come from one of the "four killer ailments" (Raghupathi, 2018):

1. Heart disease
2. Cancer
3. Diabetes
4. Alzheimer's disease

We'll be addressing all of these in Chapter 2 of this book.

7 Agers Everyone Should Know

While exploring deeper into the research of geroscience, many geroscientists point to a pioneering paper by S Jay Olshansky, which proposed that there are nine hallmarks of aging based on the cause (Olshansky, 2012). Some other scientists described aging based on the effects or processes. The bottom line is that no single factor is truly responsible for aging. These are all interdependent and also quite convoluted.

Here are seven cellular and molecular processes that model how we age from head to toe and inside out. These are the biggest players influencing the **speed and quality** of aging. They are also what I refer to throughout this book as **AGERS.**

This part will get a little more scientific, but it should still be simple enough to comprehend and take with us into the future to help us shape our own plan for taking back control of our aging process. Here are the **seven agers** we should know, including what they are and why they matter.

Ager #1 - Cellular Senescence

Len Hayflick has shown that there are limits to the number of times a cell can divide. When cells reach the limit of their ability to divide, their functions and appearance change. These altered and dysfunctional cells are known as **senescent cells**, and they become more plentiful with age (Shay 72-76). They may also appear due to other reasons, such as damage or mutation. According to the biology of humans, these senescent cells should self-destroy through a process known as **apoptosis** (self-destruction). If they do not go through apoptosis, they remain in the body as dysfunctional, take up valuable space, consume nutrients that would be more valuable to other healthy cells in the body, and secrete **senescence-associated secretory proteins (SASPs)** that trigger the inflammation in the surrounding tissue by releasing cytokines and other proinflammatory cells. This **chronic inflammation** increases the risk of four killers mentioned earlier: cancer, dementia, heart disease, and diabetes (McHugh, 2018).

When mitochondria are no longer capable of functioning, they may also release **senescence-associated mitochondrial dysfunction (SAMDs)**, which is an oxygen-reactive species that can accelerate aging at warp speed, building up over time in our tissues and organs, causing age-related slow response to the hormone insulin, which could lead to insulin resistance and type 2 diabetes. This results in the body hanging onto fat, especially around the midsection. That is why so many people get belly pouches as they age. But it's not just the belly fat we have to worry about—our organs are slowly suffocated by this fat accumulation (visceral fat), which is a far more serious problem.

When these senescent cells don't die and instead accumulate in our body, they compromise our **immune system**. This weakened immunity is why people over the age of 65 face higher risks of severe illness or death from common ailments like flu and pneumonia.

Key Things to Do to Optimize and Control Ager #1

1. There are a lot of things that we can do to prevent the barrage of senescent cells attacking our bodies. First, we want to focus on keeping the cell membranes strong for as long as possible so that cells can function properly in the first place.

2. In addition to improving our lifestyle and overall well-being, there are other things we can do. Senolytics are drugs that are designed to decrease the

number of senescent cells in the body (Hickson, Langhi Prata, et al., 2019). There have been many clinical and preclinical studies done in mice that show giving them senolytics can reduce the signs and process of aging.

3. Metformin is a common diabetes drug that is also believed to kill zombie cells in our bodies (Sunderland, Alshammarri, et al., 2023). Studies have shown that this drug can assist with many age-related disorders, including metabolic dysfunction, cardiovascular disease, cancer development, and cognitive decline. Studies also show that Metformin increases lifespan and healthspan if treatment is started early enough, although it should not be considered a "quick fix." (Mohammed, I., Hollenberg, M. D., Ding, H., & Triggle, C. R., 2021) You can talk to your doctor about it and see if it warrants consideration.

Ager #2 - Mitochondrial Dysfunction

Moving from cellular senescence to another critical aspect of aging, let's examine mitochondria—the tiny power-generating organelles in our cells. As we age, both the function and number of mitochondria decline, reducing their ability to produce energy for the cell.

Additionally, as a normal cellular functioning, cells create a natural byproduct known as reactive oxygen species (ROSs). One type of ROS is known as a **free radical**, which are unstable molecules that can damage the surrounding proteins, tissues, lipids, carbohydrates, and DNA through a process known as oxidation. Mitochondria experience free radical damage due to mutations in their own DNA, resulting in impaired energy production and cellular apoptosis. This dysfunction is linked to various health risks, including:

- Major metabolic conditions like diabetes and obesity
- Heart, kidney, liver, and gastrointestinal diseases
- Impaired hearing and vision
- Several skin conditions

In a healthy human, the free radicals are neutralized by a process known as **anti-oxidation**, which naturally happens as the body creates its own **antioxidants**. Antioxidants find free radicals in the body and bind and stabilize them. When these natural anti-oxidation processes are compromised due to aging, the oxidative stress keeps on accumulating and further damaging mitochondrial DNA and its genetic code.

Mitochondria are the power plants of the cells. When the very thing that creates the energy that keeps us alive starts to malfunction due to oxidative stress, then it's no wonder our bodies begin to fall apart, resulting in inflammation and accelerating aging throughout the body.

Key Things to Do to Optimize and Control Ager #2

Therefore, choosing a diet that is high in antioxidants and adding certain additional supplements can help fight off free radicals. Good sources of antioxidants include blueberries, dark chocolate, raspberries, spinach, tomatoes, strawberries, pecans, apples, dark leafy greens, and potatoes. We'll talk about this more later in Chapters 5 and 6.

Ager #3 - Stem Cell Exhaustion

Stem cells are the building blocks of the body. They are separated into different categories based on whether they are embryonic or adult stem cells, but they can generate (and regenerate) cells for several systems and parts of the body.

What is a stem cell? These are essentially "generic" cells that are ready to step into action and become whatever cells the body needs at the time. They exist in all parts of our bodies and can assist with everything from anti-inflammatory support to promoting the health of bones.

In the embryonic stage and in children, stem cells are typically focused on growth and development. Adult stem cells, on the other hand, primarily serve to repair and restore those cells that have been damaged. For example, if cells die in our liver, the body may send a signal to our stem cells to regenerate the lost cells to keep optimal function of the liver. Think of them like lifeguards - they essentially sit and do nothing until they are needed. When the need for more cells arises to either maintain or repair tissue due to injury or disease, they spring into action and produce new red blood cells, muscle cells, lung cells, etc., according to the need.

The problem is that there's a limited number of stem cells in each area of the body; once they are used up, they're gone.

That is called **stem cell exhaustion**. And aging doesn't make it easier; it makes it worse because these stem cells lose their capabilities as well as numbers. As this happens, the tissues in the body shrink and, eventually, will undergo atrophy.

Key Things to Do to Optimize and Control Ager #3

1. Practice Intermittent Fasting and Calories restriction as these activate autophagy, the body's natural cellular cleanup process, which supports stem cell regeneration especially in the gut and muscle tissues.

2. Both aerobic and resistance training enhances stem cell activity in the brain and muscles. Exercise also lowers chronic inflammation, creating a more favorable environment for stem cells to thrive.

3. Prioritize Quality Sleep as Restorative sleep allows stem cells to repair and regenerate. It also helps regulate hormones and reduce oxidative stress, both of which are vital for stem cell longevity.

4. Support Cellular Cleanup with Senolytics: Compounds like fisetin, quercetin (under clinical investigation) help eliminate senescent cells, which otherwise release toxic byproducts that damage the stem cell environments.

5. Boost NAD+ Levels with Supplements like NMN and NR that support mitochondrial function and DNA repair and maintain youthful stem cells.

6. Incorporate Polyphenols such as resveratrol and curcumin activate longevity pathways like sirtuins, protecting the stem cell ecosystem.

7. Consume Omega-3 Fatty Acids that helps maintain cell membrane integrity, modulate inflammatory responses and support stem cell function.

8. Hormetic Stress: Mild, controlled stressors, such as cold exposure, heat therapy, or short-term fasting help to strengthen cellular defenses and enhance stem cell resilience.

9. Adopt an Anti-Inflammatory Gut-Supportive diet rich in antioxidants, fiber, and fermented foods that helps reduce inflammation and support the gut where many adult stem cells reside.

Ager #4 - Advanced Glycation End Products (AGEs)

The next ager we will discuss is **advanced glycation end products** or **AGEs**. As we get older, our proteins, DNA, and all of the molecules in the cell cross-link, compromising the mobility and elasticity of the tissue. Through the process of **glycation**, when sugar or glucose molecules stick to the proteins, DNA, lipids, or nucleic acid, they create **AGEs**. When these AGEs accumulate, they stick together, as well as to the surrounding tissues, causing the tissue to stiffen, leading to aging signs like wrinkling of the skin, age-related cataracts, atherosclerosis in blood vessels, nephropathy, and development of Alzheimer's in the brain upon collection of Beta-amyloid. AGEs are inflammatory in nature and accelerate the aging process by creating oxidative stress in the body, finally leading to disease. When we eat food containing sugar, the glucose molecule flows through the body and binds to proteins, glycates them, and messes up the structure and function of that protein, inducing the inflammatory process in the surrounding tissue.

Key Things to Do to Optimize and Control Ager #4

Essentially, what we have to do is decrease the consumption of sugary foods or foods that can spike our blood sugar after meals. There are a lot of studies that show the harmful effects of AGEs, and these harmful effects increase with age. If we aren't managing our blood sugar and we have a constant rush of sugar throughout the body, the inflammation becomes consistent, resulting in chronic inflammation over time (Uribarri, Goodman, et al., 2010).

Ager #5 - Loss of Protein Homeostasis (Proteostasis)

Protein homeostasis, or **proteostasis**, is the process of regulating the proteins within the cells. In order for the protein molecule to do its function correctly, it must be folded perfectly into a specific shape, so it can be identified and become fully functional. If the protein's shape is distorted or not assembled right, it would not be identified accurately and will remain nonfunctional and could even become destructive.

Normally, the digestive enzyme called **lysosome** exists within the cell to neutralize and break down these dysfunctional proteins. If lysosomes are not present, then this non-functional protein would just sit in the tissue, causing toxicity in the environment and down-regulating our cells.

With age, this entire process of protein folding, as well as the function of lysosomes engulfing the distorted protein, becomes less efficient. This inefficiency leads to a lot of non-functioning proteins building up, causing problems. When lysosomes cannot keep up—either due to genetic problems or an overwhelming number of misfolded proteins—they become overworked and ineffective. This dysfunction creates a cascade of health problems. For example, it can impair blood sugar control, leading to diabetes, which in turn increases cancer risk. In the brain, when lysosomes fail to clear beta-amyloid plaques, the resulting accumulation contributes to Alzheimer's disease. Ultimately, the loss of proteostasis can create a domino effect in our bodies, leading us down a road of chronic health conditions.

Ager #6 - Telomere Shortening

Our **telomeres** are the endcaps of our DNA, which protect our chromosomes from fraying because of wear and tear. The enzyme **telomerase** is responsible for maintaining the telomeres and their length. Every time the cell divides, the telomeres keep deteriorating and shortening until they can no longer protect the cells. The cell then stops growing and undergoes apoptosis. The shortened telomeres are linked with a weakened immune system and chronic diseases like heart failure, cancer, and degenerative diseases like osteoporosis, etc.

Telomere length serves as an important indicator of health and well-being. Scientists use telomere length and their shortening rate as a biomarker to assess our biological age (how our body is aging internally) as opposed to our chronological age. People who take better care of themselves will have longer telomeres compared to their counterparts who do not exercise and do not eat well. Additionally, those with shorter than average telomeres are at higher risk for serious disease and even early death. There's also a direct connection between stress and telomere shortening (Shammas, 2011). Exercise is a great way to prevent telomere shortening. Scientists agree that even moderate exercise can significantly increase the number of longer telomeres in our bodies. At the same time, sedentary lifestyles decrease the lifespan of our telomeres and can be linked to disease and aging (Song, 2022).

Key Things to Do to Optimize and Control Ager #6

Epitalon is a synthetic peptide that works as a telomerase activator. It is modeled after a natural peptide produced by the pineal gland. When this synthetic peptide was injected into mice, it increased their lifespan by as much as 13-15%

simply because of the telomerase activation. Simultaneously, it slowed apoptosis and increased telomere lengthening (Anisimov, 2003).

A supplement called cycloastragenol has also been found to activate telomerase. Cycloastragenol is essentially a super-concentrated form of the Ayurvedic herb astragalus. Human studies of this potent supplement have shown that it can improve the biological markers associated with aging by lengthening telomeres and rescuing old cells (Yu Y, Zhou L, Yang Y, Liu Y, 2018).

Ultimately, we'll want to work on reducing our environmental and psychological stress as much as possible and get plenty of sleep so our bodies can recoup and recover accordingly.

Ager #7 - Epigenetic Changes

There are 37 trillion cells in the human body and 20,000 genes in each cell. In our genes, certain chemical compounds and proteins sit on top of our DNA and decide each cell's function. These collections of chemical compounds and proteins are called **Epigenomes**. The epigenome acts like a master key and tells our DNA when to activate a gene and when to suppress a gene, and hence controls the function of the cells. They do this by chemically marking DNA in our genome.

These epigenetic marks come in two forms: **histone acetylation** and **DNA methylation**. These are what give our cells the signal as to which function to perform and which genes to turn on or off. Epigenomes basically act as the control for cellular functioning:

- What to do
- When to do it
- Where to do it

When the process of methylation gets interfered with, accidentally certain genes turn on instead of off, or vice versa, the whole process of cellular functioning is affected. This usually happens as a result of genetic mutation due to environmental risk factors like environmental toxins, free radical exposure, radiation, gamma rays, x-rays, and environmental chemicals.

The effects of these risk factors lead to several mixed signals among the cells. When we're young and healthy, all of these biological processes are regulated within our cells. As we become older, our epigenome begins to change because of impaired histone acetylation or impaired DNA methylation. The cell cannot perform its functions and will make poor decisions, switching off and on certain genes. That, in turn, can lead to a weakened immune system, reduced muscle mass, hormone imbalances, increased risk of type 2 diabetes, increased risk of cardiovascular disease, hypertension, arteriosclerosis, and so forth.

Key Things to Do to Optimize and Control Ager #7

There are few foods that are particularly DNA methylation friendly, like green tea, salmon, spinach, avocados, and curcumin. Other categories of cruciferous vegetables like cauliflower, kale, broccoli, brussel sprouts, cabbage, turnip, and arugula are specifically very healthy for the histone acetylation process of Epigenome.

Taking Back Control Starts Now

It's never too late to add quality years to our lives. Keeping our aging population healthy and active will prevent unnecessary suffering and offset the economic burdens of older adults with multiple chronic diseases. By intervening early, we can prevent damage that would otherwise be done.

With a better understanding of the key agers involved in the aging process, we're ready to move forward into the next chapter discussing diseases of aging.

CHAPTER 2

The Role of Age-Related Diseases

Longevity is the length of one's life. Healthy aging or "healthspan" is the process of getting older while free of chronic diseases and disability. In other words, longevity describes the quantity of life, and healthspan describes the quality of life. Ideally, the two should go hand in hand.

With groundbreaking advances in medicine, the life expectancy of people around the world is increasing, leading to a rising number of aging adults. Unfortunately, this extension in longevity does not necessarily overlap with improved healthspan for the general population but instead has increased the likelihood of chronic diseases and morbidity. To be specific, according to the World Health Organization (WHO), the rise in the aging population will be accompanied by an increase in obesity, diabetes, dementia, and cancer (WHO, 2023). Therefore, understanding why aging results in progressively higher susceptibility to these life-threatening diseases has become a public health priority.

Studies show there is a direct connection between obesity, diabetes, and dementia, with obesity and diabetes contributing to a 50% increase in the risk of developing dementia (Shalev, 2017). Managing a patient with three or more of these chronic diseases is a challenging process for doctors, as well as the patients who are faced with additional struggles of lifestyle changes, quality of life, and, of course, the rising costs of healthcare.

Sadly, there is a real epidemic of chronic disease occurring among Americans. Currently, about 80% of the deaths in people over 50 years old are from heart disease, cancer, neurodegenerative disease including Alzheimer's, type 2 diabetes, and other related metabolic dysfunctions (Causes of Death, 2024).

The current medical approach to treating these age-related diseases delays mortality, but it does not prevent or reverse the decline of health. In fact, most elderly people spend the last five to eight years of their life struggling with multiple age-related diseases—each of which requires a different treatment, reducing their quality of life and crippling them financially. And who wants to experience a decreased quality of life when the "golden years" should be enjoyable, and time well spent with loved ones?

Early prevention and intervention are key. Ideally, we don't want to just live longer, but we want to live well. In order to determine how we can do that, we have to take a closer look at what is the shared mechanism among these diseases and aging.

Ultimately, Age-related Diseases Boil Down to Mitochondria Dysfunction

At the cellular level, the vast majority of age-related diseases have the same underlying cause. As we learned in Chapter 1, mitochondria are the energy factories of our cells, and their dysfunction is a key factor in aging. Over time, all of us experience some level of cellular damage, and more specifically, mitochondrial damage. Some of this damage may come from poor lifestyle choices, environmental factors, and mental stressors, and the rest is a natural effect of cellular changes throughout life.

More scientifically, our cells break down the proteins, fats, and carbohydrates in foods, also called **macronutrients**, to generate energy. Then, mitochondria use a process known as **oxidation** to convert that energy into **ATP** (adenosine triphosphate), which is the fuel that our cells store for future energy needs.

Both aging and disease damage mitochondria, disrupting their normal function and creating two problems simultaneously: they produce excess free radicals, while our aging bodies generate fewer protective antioxidants. This imbalance allows free radicals to damage surrounding cells, leading to chronic inflammation and disease. One of the most common indicators of this issue is chronic inflammation, which aggravates the aging process and often lays the groundwork for chronic diseases.

Let's take a look at five prevalent age-related diseases impacting the health span of millions of people around the world.

Age-Related Diseases

An age-related disease is one that most frequently occurs with increasing senescence. However, just because we are aging does not mean that we are destined to experience these typical age-related diseases. The following are just some of the conditions that we are at greater risk of with age.

1. Heart Disease

Heart disease is often dubbed the "silent killer" because it doesn't happen overnight. Not only that, but it creeps in virtually symptom-free. The process usually starts with **atherosclerosis** or the hardening of the heart's arteries (NIH, What Is Atherosclerosis?, 2022). Normally, a thin layer of cells called the **endothelium** protects the arterial walls. When this protective layer becomes damaged, fat molecules can penetrate the lining and build up on the walls, forming what we call **plaque**. This plaque buildup narrows the arteries, restricting blood flow to the organs and extremities. In addition to our body getting less oxygen-rich blood, our heart has to work much harder to get blood where it needs to go. This is one major cause of heart attacks, as well as angina, high blood pressure, and other cardiovascular issues.

Once the immune system becomes aware of this issue, it releases inflammatory **cytokines**, causing an **inflammatory immunological response** at the site. When the plaque dislodges and finds its way into the blood vessels of the heart and brain, it can cause a heart attack and or stroke.

Unfortunately, heart disease often comes with few warning signs or symptoms early on. The name "silent killer" was given to the disease because a startling number of people suffer severe heart attacks or strokes and even die as a result of heart-related issues with **no prior knowledge or symptoms**. This fact makes it all the more important to measure essential biomarkers through bi-annual or annual checkups. As the saying goes, *"What gets measured, gets managed."* It may not be until a patient undergoes routine diagnostic tests that an underlying heart condition may be detected. Regular measurements of the heart and arteries can help to detect the onset of heart disease that can be reversed or managed through diet, exercise, and medication where possible.

According to the American Heart Association, one person in the U.S. dies due to cardiovascular disease every **34 seconds**. Globally, heart disease is the leading killer, causing one in five deaths. In the U.S., it's one in four (Tsao, 2023). According to the World Health Organization, heart disease affects an estimated **17.9 million** lives each year (WHO, Cardiovascular Diseases, 2021). The reality is that the majority of cardiovascular diseases are preventable, whether detected or not, by reducing behavioral risks like tobacco and alcohol consumption, unhealthy diets, obesity, and physical inactivity. Ultimately, **prevention is the best defense**.

2. Diabetes

In recent decades, with the increased volume of sugar intake and the propensity for a sedentary lifestyle, the prevalence of diabetes has skyrocketed.

Type 2 diabetes is a chronic metabolic disease with insufficient response to insulin. Without insulin, the body cannot process sugar accordingly, causing excessive blood sugar levels. With the presence of chronic high blood sugar, the pancreas becomes overworked and, ultimately, no longer produces enough insulin to keep up with the body's needs, developing what is called insulin resistance (**prediabetes**). Without treatment or improvement, chronic high blood sugar leads to insulin-resistant diabetes mellitus 2.

Although the name might imply that a person is not yet faced with diabetes, prediabetes is still a sign of a very serious health risk. However, it also means that there is still time to make lifestyle changes to avoid developing full-blown diabetes.

In a well-functioning body, insulin is responsible for moving the sugar out of the blood and into the cells so that it can be converted to energy and used or stored accordingly. Those who are insulin-resistant (diabetics) cannot process sugar properly, and excess sugar causes damage to blood vessels and nerve endings, which eventually leads to serious complications like heart disease or stroke, blindness, kidney disease, and Alzheimer's.

Unfortunately, nerve damage and poor blood circulation can lead to **Peripheral Artery Disease** (PAD), causing numbness and atrophy of the affected area. As a result, some diabetics may require limbs, particularly toes, feet, or legs, to be amputated.

Diabetes can damage the endothelium in the eye's blood vessels, possibly causing total blindness due to complications. The kidneys also suffer as their filtration capabilities become damaged, leading to kidney disease/nephropathy. The brain is also impacted by chronic high blood sugar, damaging its neurons and increasing the risk of developing Alzheimer's disease.

While family history increases the risk of developing diabetes, maintaining a healthy weight can significantly reduce this risk. In fact, obesity is the number one predictor of type 2 diabetes, highlighting the critical link between these two conditions.

3. Obesity

Obesity, or the condition of having an excess amount of body fat, can have a life-threatening and often debilitating impact on the body. On a global scale, the rate of obesity has almost tripled since 1975, with more than one billion people diagnosed as obese. While 13% of all adults are obese (having a body mass index greater than 30), as many as 39% are overweight, which is equally as dangerous. Worse yet, 39 million children under the age of 5 were overweight or obese in 2020, which often sets the stage for a future of obesity, weight struggles, and chronic health issues (WHO, Obesity and Overweight, 2021).

According to a report by the World Health Organization, four million people die every year due to complications of this complex disease. While the causes of obesity may be complicated, including genetics and culture, recent changes in lifestyle and the environment have increased the likelihood of obesity.

For example, advancements in technology have decreased the need for physical activity in our daily lives, including more time sitting in cars and less time walking, and more remote processes that do not require action or movement by the user—even a remote control allows viewers to remain seated rather than getting up to change a channel. These technological advances have changed our routines, making us more sedentary and burning fewer calories.

We have also seen a dramatic increase in the consumption of highly processed foods and a decline in whole foods, including fruits, vegetables, and grains. Even fast food, although in some cases advertised as a "healthy alternative," may be loaded with preservatives, sugar, and unnecessary carbohydrates.

Medical research has definitively concluded that obesity and being overweight have a direct connection to increased risk for many of the following conditions:

- Coronary heart disease
- Type 2 diabetes
- Cancers (endometrial, breast, and colon)
- High blood pressure
- High total cholesterol
- High triglyceride levels
- Liver and gallbladder disease
- Sleep apnea and respiratory problems
- Osteoarthritis
- Stroke

The co-occurrence of diabetes and obesity has created an epidemic of global proportions. The connection here is simple, with the root cause being inflammation. The macrophages that trigger inflammation (which we will discuss in more detail in the next chapter) in the body, targeting insulin, are also causing inflammation in **adipose tissues** or our body's fat cells, causing obesity. Therefore, the more fat we have in our bodies, the more likely we are to develop insulin resistance and diabetes.

There are two kinds of fats stored in the body. Brown fat that is distributed throughout the upper back of our body is good fat. White fat, or **visceral fat**, found around the organs, can cause functionality issues due to increased inflammation when in excess.

To assess overall body composition, I recommend doing a DEXA scan, which I do bi-annually for myself as well. Essentially, it's designed to test the parameters of body fat and visceral fat, bone density, and muscle mass. Fat, muscles, and bones can all be assessed at once. It is not a dangerous or expensive test and there's minimal radiation exposure. I recommend starting these tests around age 43.

The results of the DEXA scan can provide great insight into a person's predisposition or risk of developing diabetes. For example, a low muscle mass score indicates less storage space for glucose or sugar, increasing the risk of diabetes (Alabadi B et al., 2023). Muscle mass and strength are not only essential to reduce these risks but are also essential for balance, mobility, posture, and overall longevity.

Although it is natural for the body to slow down as we age, it is also critical to maintain a healthy weight, including proper nutrition and exercise. Not only will a healthy lifestyle aid in reducing the risks of obesity and diabetes, but it also helps to lower blood pressure, reduce inflammation, decrease the risk of cancer, and lower bad (LDL) cholesterol levels.

As mentioned, diabetes and obesity go hand in hand and the benefits of maintaining a healthy lifestyle far outweigh the struggles. And I am well aware that there are temptations all around us. From advertisements of mouth-watering food to the ease of fast-food chains or processed food, the struggle is real. But to reap the rewards of longevity and increased health well into our older years, we must make real lifestyle changes, not just find the latest fad diets and trends. **Caloric restriction (CR)** and **intermittent fasting (IF)** have been found to be effective tools for losing weight, while many studies show that caloric restriction slows aging (Waziry et al., 2021).

It is also recommended to avoid grains and sugar to reduce inflammation and increase lean protein intake to develop muscle mass to make up for what we naturally lose with age.

Ultimately, following a healthy diet and remaining active have the greatest impact on avoiding obesity and possibly reversing or slowing the aging process.

4. Alzheimer's Disease

Alzheimer's Disease is a condition affecting more than 6.7 million Americans over age 65 as of 2023, and by 2050, that number is expected to rise to over 12.7 million, according to the CDC (Alzheimer's Association, 2023). Furthermore, the World Health Organization reports that more than 55 million people globally have dementia (WHO, *Dementia*, 2023).

Alzheimer's and dementia are similar, with dementia defined as any mental decline severe enough to interfere with daily life and functioning. Essentially, Alzheimer's is a specific form of dementia. Alzheimer's affects about 10% of the population over the age of 65, increasing to more than 33% among those over 85.

Microglia are special immune cells in the brain that work similarly to the body's immune cells. They are responsible for regulating the immune and inflammatory responses in the brain, as well as eliminating unhealthy neurons through a process similar to apoptosis. Microglia cells constantly monitor the brain for threats like infection or injury. When a threat is detected, they release cytokines to attack and eliminate invaders and initiate protective inflammatory response. But excessive or chronic inflammatory process can damage healthy neurons in the brain. This leads to memory loss and cognitive issues (Wang, 2020).

How does something that starts as a "mental decline" lead to death? Alzheimer's causes memory loss in its early stages, but as the disease progresses, people struggle to be aware of their surroundings or communicate effectively—typically living up to 4 to 8 years after diagnosis.

One reason Alzheimer's is deadly is that people lose the ability to properly swallow food and drinks. In addition to nutritional deficiencies, this increases the risk of food getting into the lungs, leading to infection and pneumonia. According to UCLA Health, **aspiration pneumonia** is the leading cause of death among patients (Ask the Doctors - What is the cause of death in Alzheimer's disease? 2018). Some patients may even inhale gastric fluids.

Many suffering from Alzheimer's and dementia also die due to accidents, such as falling down stairs or going outside unsupervised. Other common reasons that people die include dehydration leading to kidney failure, increased isolation and changes in routine care causing bedsores and sepsis, malnutrition resulting in a lack of immunity, and infections.

Routine screening to test for brain amyloids is an effective tool to detect Alzheimer's. Scientists have also created a blood test that is 96% accurate at predicting Alzheimer's in younger patients. A genetic predisposition can be determined via DNA testing, which looks for **APP amyloid precursor genes** PSEN1 and PSEN2 (NAG, 2023).

As with the rest of the diseases here, we'll talk more in-depth about what we can do later. For now, know that exercise, proper sleep, nutrition, and **intellectual stimulation** are important in maintaining brain health. Engaging in crosswords, sudoku, puzzles, logic puzzles, reading, bingo, and other brain-working activities helps as well.

As for treatment options, studies are being done on anti-amyloid beta vaccines, but they're still very early in development. More often, people consider plasma infusions, red light therapy, and hyperbaric oxygen therapies to assist in warding off inflammation. Correcting the gut microbiome reduces inflammation and less neuroinflammation means a dramatic reduction in amyloids.

5. Cancer

According to the National Cancer Institute, 39.5% of people are diagnosed with cancer in their lifetime and 1.73 million people are diagnosed with cancer each year. By 2040, the number of new cancer cases per year is expected to rise to 29.5 million per year as life expectancy increases (NCI, 2023).

The origin of cancer cells and their growth is primarily due to DNA damage and cell mutation. The primary cause of mutated cells and damaged DNA is free radical accumulation and oxidative stress brought upon by dysfunctional mitochondria. When the mitochondria become dysfunctional, typically because of aging, they aren't capable of producing enough energy, creating an ideal environment for the creation of cancer cells. The immune system also weakens with age, causing dysregulation in homeostasis/balance, adding to the risk of cancer cell growth.

Some believe that cancer is solely a genetic problem. However, the data shows that only two to five percent of cancers are genetically based (Anand, 2008). The rest are caused by mitochondrial dysfunction. This theory is based on the concept that the affected mitochondria undergo **anaerobic metabolism**. This means they switch from their energy-producing oxidation mode (presence of oxygen) to burning carbohydrates (without oxygen.) The vast majority of cancers are associated with anaerobic metabolism. Therefore, keeping our mitochondria strong drastically reduces our cancer risk.

Activating **autophagy** (the body's natural detox process and cleansing to remove the damaged cells and their cellular components from the body), reducing inflammation, and boosting mitochondrial health are three strong defenses, along with specific supplements and lifestyle modifications. Combining all of these modalities helps to improve overall aging, increase longevity, and reduce the risk of age-related diseases. We will talk about all of these healthspan-increasing options in the following chapters.

Improving Our Chances Against Chronic Diseases Due to Aging

The aging process is inevitable; however, we do not have to be resigned to those years being filled with chronic disease, distress, and unhappiness. Longevity and increased lifespan can include improved healthspan but it will require work.

The following are several suggestions for living a lifestyle that will reduce our risk of developing many of the chronic diseases described above, as well as increasing our chances of living a healthy, fulfilling life well into our older years.

1. Caloric restriction (CR) and intermittent fasting (IF) serve dual purposes: controlling unwanted weight gain and speeding up stem cell regeneration, which helps rejuvenate the body's tissues.

2. Eating a wide variety of fruits and vegetables rich in vitamins C & E, as well as supplements containing antioxidants to fight off oxidative damage in the body.

3. Restricting or avoiding saturated fats and trans fats, adding intake of Omega-3 supplements, and eating foods rich in polyunsaturated fats helps to keep inflammation under control.

4. Restricting as much sugar and processed foods as possible to avoid advanced glycosylation end products (AGEs).

5. Cook meats using moist heat, and low temperature with shorter cooking times, and marinating with lemon, vinegar, and tomatoes helps to reduce glycation end products.

6. Sweating by high-intensity intervals (HIIT), as well as strength training helps the body to produce more antioxidants and boost mitochondria, reducing the risk of age-related diseases.

7. Sleeping a full eight hours is non-negotiable to heal, repair, and detoxify.

Even though such age-related diseases appear unavoidable, insight into the biological processes that govern aging will allow us to find effective prevention or postponement of them. In the following chapter, we will elaborate on these underlying processes in greater detail.

CHAPTER 3

Three Core Processes That Age Us

Aging is a multifactorial complex phenomenon manifested at the genetic, molecular, cellular, organ, and system levels due to the consequences of gradual wear and tear on the body over time, which results in an increased risk of diseases and a reduction in lifespan (Guo,2022).

Three harmful biological processes are going on inside the body as we age, making us more susceptible to chronic diseases of aging, i.e., diabetes, obesity, cardiovascular disease, Alzheimer's, and cancers, and diminishing our capacity to withstand environmental/internal physiological toxicity (Liguori, 2018).

To better understand how to slow or reverse the damage caused by aging and the risk of these age-related diseases, it is important to first thoroughly understand these three processes that wreak havoc in our bodies and ultimately reduce our health and lifespan:

1. Oxidation
2. Inflammation
3. Decreased ability for detoxification

3 Harmful Biological Processes of Aging

Oxidation

The first internal process of aging occurs when free radicals/reactive oxygen species (ROS) accumulate at high levels, causing oxidative stress in surrounding tissues (Warraich, 2020). While ROS are normal byproducts of cellular energy generation, their excessive accumulation damages critical cellular components, including lipids, nucleic acids, proteins, DNA, and mitochondria. These oxidative modifications cause substantial physiological impact by altering the structure and function of essential biological molecules.

Besides endogenous ROS, there are massive external triggers that also contribute to oxidation, which include UV radiation, pathogens, and environmental toxins like herbicides, insecticides, and heavy metals.

This endogenous and exogenous oxidative damage leads to diseases and age-related complications.

Inflammation

The second process of aging is inflammation. This phenomenon typically occurs with age and is characterized by chronic, low-grade inflammation (Salminen, 2013), which has been referred to as "inflammaging" (Ferrucci, 2018). This persistent inflammation Subsequently increases the risk of age-related diseases such as cardiovascular and chronic kidney diseases, diabetes, cancer, depression, dementia, and sarcopenia.

With age, senescent cells accumulate in multiple tissues, causing biological and functional decline. Cellular senescence is a biological process where cells stop dividing and secrete proinflammatory molecules called 'senescence-associated secretory protein' (SASP), which are highly inflammatory and trigger chronic systemic inflammation.

This chronic inflammation is believed to result from a combination of triggering factors such as:

1. Genetic Susceptibility: Changes in gene expression (DNA damage, telomere shortening, mitochondrial dysfunction, epigenetic changes) with age can contribute to chronic inflammation.

2. Central Obesity: Excess fat, especially around the abdomen, can produce pro-inflammatory compounds that contribute to inflammation.

3. Altered Gut Permeability: Changes in the gut microbiota and increased intestinal permeability can lead to the leakage of bacteria and toxins into the bloodstream, triggering an immune response and inflammation.

4. Cellular Senescence: Senescent cells, which have stopped dividing and acquired a pro-inflammatory secretory profile, can contribute to systemic inflammation.

5. Oxidative Stress: Dysfunctional mitochondria and increased oxidative stress can trigger inflammatory responses.

6. Immune Cell Dysregulation: Changes in immune cell function and regulation can lead to chronic inflammation.

Decreased ability for detoxification

As we age, oxidative damage progressively accumulates in our cells. Simultaneously, our body's natural detoxification system becomes less efficient. The key enzyme in this process—glutathione transferase (GST)—gradually loses its ability to clear away oxidative byproducts. This dual problem—more damage combined with reduced cleaning capacity—severely compromises our body's ability to detoxify itself.

The reduction of glutathione transferase activity with age is attributed to several factors, like a decline in enzyme production and nutritional deficiencies, such as:

1. Glutathione precursors (e.g., cysteine, glutamine, glycine)
2. Vitamins (e.g., vitamins C and E)
3. Minerals (e.g., selenium)

Also, when oxidative damage is out of control, our lysosomes or lysosomal proteins (the body's inbuilt detoxification through lymphatics) become inefficient at clearing the toxins out of the body.

And altogether, this whole cycle contributes to increased susceptibility to premature aging and various chronic health issues such as immunodeficiency, cancer, and neurodegenerative diseases.

Key Things to Do to Optimize and Control These Processes of Aging

Although oxidation, inflammation, and impaired detoxification are inevitable results of aging, we are not powerless against these processes. Through targeted intervention, we can effectively reverse these processes to a large extent and maintain our health. Let us examine some measures that counteract each of the three mechanisms of aging. These measures aim to lessen inflammation, fight oxidation, and enhance detoxification.

1. Chronic stress is damaging to the body and brain as well. It alters our circadian rhythm and increases inflammation and insulin resistance. Try to reduce your day-to-day stress at all costs.

2. Regulate your sleep and wake cycle. Get full-spectrum sunlight in the morning and limit your exposure to blue and bright light at night.

3. Eat your vegetable and fruit servings per day, which contain tons of polyphenols and anti-inflammatory substances. Avoid refined carbohydrates, sugar, and trans-fat (vegetable oil, seed oil, and rancid oil, which are high in omega-6 fatty acids). These foods overwhelm our bodies with chronic inflammation and contribute to heart disease. Instead of vegetable oil, I recommend cooking with fruit oil (olive oil or avocado oil).

4. Eat fatty fish and seafood (rich sources of EPA/DHA) and supplement with 1.5 grams of Omega-3 fatty acid per day in the form of a pill.

5. Exercise and intermittent fasting increase the body's ability to detoxify and boost autophagy (the body's process of getting rid of dead and damaged cells) and mitophagy (the body's process of getting rid of dead and damaged mitochondria), thus reducing overall inflammation and oxidation.

6. Consume antioxidant-rich food, supplements of vitamin C and vitamin E, and eat one Brazil nut every day (daily serving of selenium).

7. Monitor High-sensitivity C-reactive protein (hs-CRP) which is an indicator of inflammation. If your hs-CRP is greater than 0.5, that is an indication of a low-level chronic inflammation.

8. Adding a tablespoon of apple cider vinegar to a glass of water before meals can help lower blood sugar levels, particularly before carbohydrate-rich foods. This simple remedy works by activating the AMPK pathway—similar to how the diabetes medication Metformin functions. Research supports its effectiveness for weight management as well; a 2014 study found that people following a low-calorie diet who added apple cider vinegar before meals lost significantly more weight than those following the same diet without vinegar.

9. If you struggle with non-clinical blood sugar rises or if the diabetes treatment medication metformin is contraindicated for a certain reason, try a blood sugar-lowering supplement like berberine, 500 milligrams, two times daily. Also, try cinnamon, which helps to lower the blood sugar level.

10. Take a daily dose of CoQ10, an antioxidant for cardiovascular health.

11. Take a daily dose of Lutein and Zeaxanthin, antioxidants for the eyes.

12. Glutathione is a major antioxidant in our body. I regularly supplement intramuscular (IM) 600-1200 milligrams once a month and take liposomal glutathione daily for better delivery.

13. I supplement combined glycine and NAC (N-acetylcysteine, a precursor of glutathione synthesis) nightly.

14. I supplement activated charcoal for a month, four times per year. Because of its adsorption properties, it binds all the heavy metals and toxins and detoxifies them out of the body.

15. Sweating through saunas/HIIT exercises helps eliminate toxins through the skin and lessens the burden of heavy metals out of our body.

CHAPTER 4

The Hidden Impact of Environmental And Mental Stressors

All around us lie stressors and toxins that impact the body, causing premature aging and chronic ailments. From morning to evening and even while we sleep, our bodies are exposed to insidious contaminants that infiltrate our systems. These toxins affect our immune function, damage our mitochondria, and accelerate cellular deterioration—directly impacting the aging processes we discussed in previous chapters.

From environmental factors to mental stressors, everything in our daily lives has an impact on our physical well-being, overall health, and longevity.

Environmental stressors

Let's consider some of the stressors that impact our health from the moment we wake up. For example, the air in our house may contain airborne pollutants like dust, mold spores, volatile organic compounds (VOCs) from household cleaners, fabric fibers, and pet dander. The water we use to brush our teeth from the tap may contain chlorine, chloramines, and potentially heavy metals, including lead, mercury, and cadmium. The shampoos, soaps, toothpaste, cosmetics, creams, lotions, and other skincare products could possibly be made of parabens, phthalates, triclosan, and formaldehyde-releasing agents. And all of this before breakfast!

The food we eat has been processed and packaged while being exposed to pesticides, artificial colors, preservatives (BHT, BHA), Bisphenol A (BPA), and phthalates.

During our commute to work and in our daily work environment, we may be exposed to vehicle emissions, including nitrogen dioxide (NO_2), sulfur dioxide (SO_2), and carbon monoxide (CO).

Computers, printers, and cell phones expose us to potentially harmful electromagnetic radiation.

The soaps, sanitizers, and detergents used in general cleaning may expose us to high levels of ammonia, bleach, and other harsh chemicals.

Many people use non-stick cookware in their homes, which can release harmful toxins such as perfluorooctanoic acid (PFOA), and gas stoves can emit nitrogen dioxide (NO_2).

VOCs from paint, furniture, carpets, and electronic devices may also be present, especially in homes with poor ventilation, leading to higher concentrations of indoor air pollutants.

Although many of us consider pollutants and toxins to be external to our home, what about those things that impact us even while we sleep, such as mattresses, pillows, and bedding, which can off-gas chemicals like formaldehyde and flame retardants and can harbor dust mites and allergens.

Heavy metals such as lead, mercury (often found in seafood), arsenic, and cadmium (found in tobacco smoke) disrupt mitochondrial functioning and damage DNA. Heavy metal contaminants are often found in old paint, contaminated soil, and unfiltered drinking water.

Microplastics can be ingested through food and water or inhaled from the air. Also, organic pollutants (POPs) produced in agriculture and industrial manufacturing are released into the atmosphere, affecting the water supply and food chain.

Electromagnetic radiation, exposing our eyes and brain to blue light from electronic devices, can interfere with sleep patterns and melatonin production.

Mercury from amalgam fillings and fluoride-containing toothpaste are the toxic additives in dental procedures and oral care that impact cell mutation.

Prescription antibiotics impact our digestive health and immunity by killing good bacteria along with bad bacteria in the gut, causing impaired digestion and, hence, nutritional deficiencies.

Scientific Basis – Environmental Factors' Impact on our Bodies

The question is, what is the impact of these environmental toxins on our bodies?

Environmental pollutants can cause health problems like respiratory diseases, heart disease, and some types of cancer

(Brusseau et al., 2019), including chronic diseases. The accumulation of toxic chemicals and pollutants in the body's systems can lead to immune dysfunction, autoimmunity, asthma, allergies, cancers, cognitive deficit, mood changes, neurological illnesses, changes in libido, reproductive dysfunction, and glucose dysregulation (Crinnion, 2000).

Let's look at the biological impact of some of the environmental stressors we discussed previously:

1. Air pollutants like nitrogen dioxide (NO2), sulfur dioxide (SO2), and ozone (O3) penetrate the respiratory system and enter the bloodstream, where they cause oxidative damage affecting lipids, proteins, and DNA, causing subsequent inflammation and cellular damage.

2. Heavy metals such as lead, mercury, arsenic, and cadmium disrupt mitochondrial function and hence alter DNA and gene expression, contributing to premature aging. Lead exposure can cause permanent intellectual disabilities, behavioral disorders, and delays in puberty.

3. Chlorine and chloramines found in cleaning and disinfecting products induce apoptosis, causing cellular death and increased risk of certain cancers.

4. Fluoride, commonly used to prevent cavities, causes oxidative damage to DNA and, hence, alters cellular function.

5. Pesticides and Herbicides contain glyphosates, which simulate hormones and, hence, block hormone receptors, disrupting endocrine functioning and causing reproductive and metabolic disorders (U.S. Department of Health, 2016).

6. Phthalates used in personal care products are known endocrine disruptors, leading to reproductive and developmental issues. Parabens, which are preservatives found in cosmetics and personal care products, bind to estrogen receptors, causing oxidative damage to estrogen and, hence, contributing to breast cancer risk. Formaldehyde, a known carcinogen found in various personal care products, forms crosslinks within proteins, altering their function and leading to cellular dysfunction.

7. Bisphenol A (BPA), found in plastics, is an endocrine disruptor that binds to estrogen receptors. It disrupts hormonal balance and leads to metabolic and reproductive issues.

Mental stressors

While environmental toxins attack our bodies from the outside, psychological stress damages us from within. Life is stressful, and we are exposed to circumstances and situations that create the perfect situation for this stress to have a negative impact on our bodies.

Common mental stressors include illness, injury, major life changes (marriage, divorce, childbirth), parenting challenges, and work/home pressures. These stressors trigger the release of cortisol and adrenaline—hormones that disrupt circadian rhythms, increase inflammation, elevate insulin resistance and blood glucose levels, and redirect energy from digestion and reproduction to muscles and brain for "fight or flight" responses. In all these scenarios, the body assumes that you are going through a fight or flight mechanism/sympathetic nervous system regulation, causing an accumulation of furthermore cortisol that sets the stage for chronic inflammation, oxidative stress, and hormonal imbalances disrupting cellular homeostasis.

When mental and environmental stress superimpose, they create a synergistic effect that increases the vulnerability of cells to environmental toxins, thereby intensifying the risk of age-related diseases such as cardiovascular disease, neurodegenerative disorders, and cancer. Studies show that up to 70% of chronic diseases and premature aging can be attributed to the interplay between mental and environmental stress. This explains the importance of addressing both psychological and environmental well-being as part of a holistic approach to health and longevity (Pu, 2024).

Scientific Basis – Mental Stressors' Impact on our Bodies

The impact of mental stress has far-reaching long-term effects on our cells, mitochondria, and DNA.

1. Chronic stress leads to the overproduction of free radicals and reactive oxygen species (ROS), which cause oxidative damage to cells and mitochondria, further imbalancing cellular homeostasis and causing cellular death (apoptosis).

2. Telomeres, which are protective caps at the ends of chromosomes, are shortened due to chronic stress, triggering cellular senescence and leading to premature cellular aging.

3. Chronic stress also increases the incidence of altered gene expression on DNA and increases the risk of cancer.

4. Cortisol, the primary stress hormone, has several long-term effects on the body, including immune suppression, insulin resistance, breakdown of muscle protein, and the storage of fat, particularly in the abdominal area, contributing to obesity and metabolic syndrome.

Even though stress in the right amount is perfectly normal and critical for survival, chronic elevation of the catecholamines, adrenaline, and norepinephrine can have detrimental effects, like cardiovascular, neurodegenerative, and cognitive decline.

Key Things to Do

Lifestyle, personal habits and behaviors, social connections, and reduced exposure to environmental toxins can support our bodies to cleanse, defend, and thrive in day-to-day life.

Lifestyle and Environmental Modifications

1. Air/water Quality Improvement

- Use HEPA air purifiers to reduce indoor air pollutants such as dust, pollen, and VOCs.
- Ensure proper ventilation in your home to reduce the concentration of indoor pollutants. Use exhaust fans in kitchens and bathrooms.
- Install high-quality water filters (e.g., activated carbon filters or reverse osmosis systems) to remove contaminants such as chlorine, heavy metals, and pesticides.
- Periodical testing of your water supply for contaminants.
- Use BPA-free bottled water or glass containers to avoid plastic chemicals like BPA.
- Use glass or stainless steel containers for food and beverages instead of plastic.

2. Personal Care Products

- Opt for natural and organic personal care products free from parabens, phthalates, and formaldehyde-releasing agents.

- Carefully read product labels and avoid ingredients known to be harmful.

3. Household Cleaning

- Use eco-friendly/green cleaning products that do not contain harsh chemicals.
- Make your own cleaning solutions using natural ingredients like vinegar, baking soda, and lemon juice.
- Opt for natural pest control methods and avoid chemical pesticides.

4. Sustainable Living

- Choose organic produce and buy from local farmers to reduce exposure to pesticides, herbicides, and long-term storage chemicals.

5. Antioxidant-Rich Foods

- Consume a variety of colorful fruits and vegetables, such as berries, leafy greens, and cruciferous vegetables.
- Include nuts and seeds, like almonds, walnuts, and flaxseeds.
- Incorporate herbs and spices like turmeric, ginger, and garlic.

6. Hydration

- Drink plenty of purified water to help flush out toxins from the body.

- Consume herbal teas that support detoxification, like green tea, dandelion root tea, and chamomile.

7. Antioxidants

- Supplements like Vitamin C, Vitamin E, Glutathione, and Coenzyme Q10 are powerful antioxidants that help to neutralize free radicals and support detoxification.

8. Detoxification Support

- Milk Thistle: Supports liver function and detoxification.
- N-Acetylcysteine (NAC): A precursor to glutathione, helps in detoxification.
- Activated Charcoal binds to toxins and heavy metals and helps with their elimination.

Lifestyle Behaviors

1. Physical Activity

- Regular physical activity such as walking, jogging, running, cycling, and swimming boost endorphin levels, improve mood, and reduce stress (Childs, 2014).
- Lifting weights/strength training helps to reduce stress by improving physical strength, boosting endorphins, and providing a sense of accomplishment.

- Yoga, breathing exercises, and meditation reduce stress by promoting relaxation.
- Sweat through saunas/HIIT exercises to help eliminate toxins through the skin.

2. Stress Management

- Practice mindfulness, meditation, or deep breathing exercises to reduce stress.
- Prioritize sleep to get no less than seven and no more than nine hours per night.
- Maintain a healthy circadian rhythm by regulating your sleep and wake cycle, getting full-spectrum sunlight in the morning, limiting exposure to blue light at night, keeping a consistent sleep schedule, blocking out all light and sounds in your bedroom, tracking sleep consistently using gadgets like aura ring and reducing the consumption of caffeine and alcohol in the evening.
- Maintaining strong social ties, engaging in meaningful conversations, journaling your thoughts, engaging in painting, music, or crafting, and organizing your day-to-day time can provide a mental break and reduce stress.

Supplements to Reduce Mental Stress

- Adaptogens like ashwagandha, rhodiola rosea, and holy basil help to lower cortisol levels and improve overall well-being.

- Omega-3 Fatty Acids found in fish oil support brain health and have been shown to reduce symptoms of anxiety and depression.

- Magnesium helps to reduce anxiety and promote calm.

- L-Theanine found in green tea promotes relaxation without causing drowsiness.

- GABA (Gamma-Aminobutyric Acid), a neurotransmitter, helps to promote relaxation and reduce anxiety by inhibiting neural activity.

- Valerian Root, traditionally used in Eastern medicine, helps to promote relaxation and improve sleep quality.

- B Vitamins, particularly B6, B9 (folate), and B12, support the nervous system, reduce stress, and improve mood.

- Probiotics: Gut health is linked to mental health. Probiotics improve gut microbiome, which in turn helps to reduce anxiety and improve mood.

CHAPTER 5

Lifestyle, Supplements, And Longevity Connection

Supplements can help with health and aging, but do not expect them to do all the work or make up for unhealthy practices. When added to a healthy diet and lifestyle, supplements can enhance overall health and well-being.

According to the NHANES survey published by the CDC, a large percentage of Americans' diets are deficient in critical micronutrients—94% do not get enough Vitamin D, 53% do not get enough magnesium, and 44% do not get enough calcium (CDC 2024). For some people, diets that contain a lot of processed foods and lack diversity of fruits and vegetables can cause deficiencies. While for some others, even those who eat a healthy whole-food diet or minimally processed foods (with an emphasis on a variety of colorful plants) can still come up short on certain nutrients because of declining soil quality and inadequate nutrient absorption.

There are plenty of opinions out there on supplements. Some experts say they are essential, and others say they are unnecessary. Navigating all of the options can get confusing. I try to keep it simple. As a baseline, I take supplements for nutrients that are difficult to get from food alone (and naturally lacking in most people). I use supplements with two strategies.

1. Baseline Supplements: These cover the most common nutritional deficiencies that affect nearly everyone in our modern world.
2. Specialty Supplements: These target specific body systems or address personal health goals based on individual needs.

Supporting metabolic health requires a combination of healthy nutrition, physical activity, stress reduction, restorative sleep, optimizing circadian rhythm, and selecting supplementation as needed.

Before starting any supplement regimen, I recommend testing to identify your specific deficiencies. However, if testing isn't feasible, the basic supplements I'll outline can still be beneficial for most people. Regular measurement of key biomarkers, ideally twice yearly, allows us to adapt and adjust the supplement protocol based on the body's changing needs. If you have specific health complications, more frequent testing may be necessary, as directed by your healthcare provider.

Omega-3s, vitamin D, magnesium, B-complex, and minerals complex are useful for general daily health maintenance to optimize cellular health and aging. Deficiencies in these nutrients are commonly discovered based on laboratory testing for most people. I always like to test ferritin levels in men and women because it is a marker of iron storage. Iron is the mineral that allows our red blood cells to carry oxygen, which mitochondria need for cellular respiration. If ferritin is low (<75 ng/mL), I recommend supplementing with iron. If ferritin is high (>150 ng/mL), this can cause oxidative stress. In that case, I advise donating blood to lower their iron loads.

Gut Dysfunctions

Pesticides, herbicides, poor nutrition, prescription drugs, antibiotics, and industrial farming all destroy the healthy bacteria in the gut, which is essential for good health. Those with gut dysfunctions have impaired nutrient absorption and will have problems with hormone imbalance, compromised immunity, brain fog, bloating, skin issues, and fungal infections due to the overgrowth of bad bacteria. This happens as a result of inflammation/leaky gut, even when we eat wholesome and healthy foods.

As a result of inflammation and leaky gut, toxins, and digestive end products cross the gut membrane and enter our bloodstream where they do not belong. Our body will do anything to get them out, and one of the ways it does is through the skin. This can lead to a myriad of skin issues like acne, psoriasis, dermatitis, eczema, sagging and wrinkled skin, blemishes, and blisters. Because of compromised immunity, those with these issues will have symptoms of food allergies and intolerance. For those with skin issues, food allergies, or bloating, we need to focus on treating and healing the gut with probiotics, chlorophyll, minerals, and omega-3 fatty acids.

Gut healing and recovery are very important. It can take up to three months to start seeing results. I like to source my probiotic needs from natural food sources by consuming fermented foods like kimchi, sauerkraut, kvass, kefir, and unsweetened yogurt. In some severe cases of gut dysfunction and dysbiosis, it might be necessary to add high-quality, live-culture probiotics to the protocol and follow an elimination diet.

Collagen

Collagen is the most abundant protein in our body, and it acts as a building block for our bones, teeth, muscles, skin, and other connective tissues. Research shows that collagen supplements improve skin elasticity, reduce wrinkles, boost skin hydration, and increase the density of fibroblasts (the cells in connective tissue) (Al-Atif, 2022). Supplementing with collagen is a must because collagen production slows down as we get older. After the age of 25, we break down more collagen than we build, and this is often when we begin to see our first fine lines and wrinkles. From there, we start losing about 1% of our collagen each year. Excess sun exposure, smoking, and too much UV light exposure all degrade collagen even more quickly.

Collagen protein powders are usually hydrolyzed, meaning they have been partially broken down into the main amino acids hydroxyproline and other peptides. The body needs sufficient vitamin C to produce collagen and maintain its vitality. Therefore, always read the label to ensure the terms hydrolyzed collagen and added vitamin C are in the ingredient list for appropriate bioavailability.

Collagen supplements do other things as well. They reduce joint pain and boost the density of our cartilage, making joints more flexible. Collagen also repairs and strengthens the intestinal and stomach lining. The amino acid **glycine**, which makes up a third of collagen, also helps our body produce more stomach acid, which aids in digestion and reduces acid reflux. Glycine is actually an inhibitory neurotransmitter, which helps to calm the nervous system to get better quality sleep.

Toxin Avoidance & Detox

One of the most important things we can do to optimize cellular function is to avoid toxins that directly damage cellular DNA and contribute to aging. These are listed below:

- Household mold exposure
- Alcohol
- Certain drugs (e.g., antibiotics, acetaminophen, cocaine, amphetamine, NSAIDs, and statins)
- Heavy metals (e.g., mercury, arsenic, cadmium, and lead)
- Phthalates and parabens in beauty products
- Pesticides
- Persistent contaminants in unfiltered tap water
- Excessive EMF

In people who have been exposed to metal toxicity, an active detoxification protocol with EDTA chelation therapy (Filippo, 2022) and activated charcoal may be required under the supervision of an expert. IV Glutathione helps efficiently detox from heavy metals, as glutathione is one of the body's most powerful antioxidants (Jozefczak, 2012) and a natural chelating agent. I am a huge fan of IV Glutathione and get it done regularly (two times per year). In addition, I also take an oral dose of high-quality glutathione daily, preferably before using an infrared sauna, for the added benefits of detoxification. The brand I am using is Cymbiotica, which is committed to its high-quality products with a liposomal delivery system.

I follow a 4-week detox cycle with active charcoal 3 - 4 times per year. This approach effectively helps eliminate heavy metals, such as cadmium, copper, nickel, and lead, that may accumulate in the body over time. Detoxifying the heavy metals out of the body helps support a healthy digestive system, kidney, and liver. While detoxing with activated charcoal, try not to eat meals or take any other supplementation within a 2-hour window before and after, as it can bind to prescription medicine, vitamins, supplements, and nutrients in the food and nullify their effects due to its strong binding nature. Try to consume a lot of water while detoxifying, as hydration is a must to flush toxins out of the system.

Additionally, I drink a glass of water with a few chlorophyll drops first thing in the morning. Chlorella is one of the greatest superfoods on the planet. It is high in protein and B vitamins and is a mega detoxifier. Scientists have researched chlorella extensively and have found that it binds with mercury in the gut. It is generally a very good practice to consume chlorella if fish is a regular part of our diet (Rafati-Rahimzadeh, 2014).

Stay Hydrated

On average, the body loses 2-3 quarts of water per day. These fluids need replacing for bodily function, so hydration is essential. The best source of hydration is water. Water is a game changer for our body, brain, and skin, which looks plumper and fresher when we are hydrated. Every morning, I like to add lemon juice to my glass of water to cleanse, alkalize, and boost immunity.

Ideally, women should drink 11.5 cups (2.7 liters), and men should drink 15.5 cups (3.7 liters) of water per day, according to the U.S. National Academies of Sciences, Engineering, and Medicine (U.S. National Academies of Sciences, Engineering, and Medicine, 2005).

One simple way to calculate our daily water intake in ounces is to aim for half our body weight in pounds each day to stay well hydrated. It is a good practice to add a pinch of Celtic salt to our water as it improves the efficiency of hydration. Celtic salt, through the process of osmosis, pulls all the water that we drink into our cells and keeps them hydrated.

Daily Basic Supplements

Vitamin/Supplement	What It Does	Dose
Vitamin D-3 + K-2	D-3 - Anti-inflammatory benefits. Improves immunity, brain health, and bone density. K-2 - Promotes the calcification of bone and reduces calcium deposits in blood vessels.	D-3: 5000 IU Once Daily K-2: 100 mcg Daily
Omega 3 Fatty Acids (DHA, EPA)	Anti-inflammatory supports brain, heart, skin, and hair health. DHA promotes brain function, and EPA is good for heart health.	1000 mg Daily
Iodine in the form of Potassium Iodine	High Potency Iodine is an essential element supporting thyroid health.	12.5 mg Daily
Zinc & Selenium	Zinc - Improves immune health and overall wellness. Selenium is an antioxidant and an essential trace mineral that supports normal thyroid function and optimal metabolic health.	15 mg of Zinc 200 mcg of Selenium
Electrolytes & Minerals	A balanced intake of electrolytes and minerals is vital for maintaining the body's electrical and physiological function.	Besides optimal intake of food, added supplementation is required since modern-day soil and farming are deficient in providing nutrients in our food. * Sodium, potassium, iron, zinc, copper,

		magnesium, iodine, and selenium ** Chloride helps maintain fluid balance and is a part of stomach acid (HCl). *** Bicarbonates as a buffer to maintain acid-base balance for metabolic processes.
Vitamin C	Supports immunity and antioxidant benefits.	1000 mg Daily
Magnesium (Mg)	Magnesium is involved in over 300 biochemical processes in the body, making it essential for overall well-being. Crucial for optimal brain and nerve health, contributing to cognitive functions, mood regulation, and modulating stress and anxiety.	A combination of topical Magnesium citrate and oral Magnesium threonate - 1000 - 2000 MG, which provides about 200 - 250 mg of elemental Magnesium. ** Magnesium threonate is the only form of Mg that can cross the blood-brain barrier (BBB).
Creatine	Creatine stores and donates phosphate molecules to ADP to regenerate ATP (primary energy carrier). Creatine's primary role in energy production is to improve exercise performance, build muscle mass, and prevent muscle injury.	3-5 g daily, depending on an individual's need (athletic intensity). There is no specific time of intake, but I generally take my creatine dose before or after workouts.
Hydrolyzed Collagen	Promotes strong bones, joints, and teeth, leaner muscles, and healthy skin.	10 mg daily

Grass-fed Whey Protein Powder w/ branch-chain amino acids (Containing Leucine, Isoleucine, Valine)	To meet daily protein needs to improve muscle health, immune health, and overall wellness.	25-30 g per serving dose If vegetarian, then look for hemp, pea, or pumpkin seed sourced and avoid soy.
Melatonin	Melatonin is a hormone naturally secreted by the pineal gland that stimulates and regulates sleep. The brain's natural melatonin production is far superior (e.g., dimming the lights, consistent sleeping time, minimizing screen time, and using a pair of red lens glasses after sunset to support the body's natural circadian rhythm).	Use only if needed to optimize sleep quantity and quality. 5 mg or as suggested by your physician 30 - 60 minutes before bedtime
Probiotics	Get probiotics as much as possible from natural foods, such as Kimchi, Sauerkraut, Kvass, Kefir, and Unsweetened Yogurt. Supplement with high-quality live culture probiotic supplements if needed or per your personal choice. Promising new research suggests that consuming probiotic-rich fermented foods may be a better option than supplements (Soemarie, 2021)	
Fiber	Fiber is essential to feeding our gut microbiome, which	

	then produces beneficial metabolites—short-chain fatty acids that improve insulin sensitivity and decrease inflammation. However, skip the fiber supplements, which may contain sugar and artificial colors and flavors. Fiber from whole plants is far superior. Aim for 30-50 grams of fiber per day from sources like chia seeds, flax seeds, avocados, beans, lentils, and berries.	
Calcium	Excessive calcium through unmonitored supplementation may cause plaque build-up in the arteries (Morelli, 2020) Aim to get the daily calcium requirement from food sources such as dairy products, sardines (with bones), almonds, tahini, and dark leafy greens (cooked to reduce oxalates, which can inhibit calcium absorption).	

Lifestyle

Lifestyle improvements are undoubtedly a major factor in aging. Over the years, we expose our bodies to a variety of substances either inadvertently (environmental toxins and general wear and tear) or on purpose (smoking, alcohol, late-night sleep, and unhealthy food choices). Making lifestyle changes now can have a direct effect on our future in terms of aging and avoiding chronic diseases.

Infrared Light

Red/infrared light therapy uses different wavelengths of light to restore, repair, and protect tissue that is injured and degenerating as we age while also improving mitochondrial function by activating stem cells. Infrared light increases nitric oxide levels, an important molecule our body produces that keeps blood vessels healthy. More nitric oxide increases circulation, which ensures that all of our cells are nourished by blood, oxygen, and nutrients. Infrared light therapy effectively treats muscle fatigue and injuries, the reason that keeps many people from exercising as they age.

Spending time in a sauna (infrared or not) also leads our body to produce **heat shock proteins** (HSPs), which prevent protein degradation caused by oxidative stress, remove free radicals, and boost glutathione levels. I use infrared saunas regularly (3 - 4 times a week for 25 minutes each session) for general detoxification. I enjoy using my Sunlighten M pulse sauna unit at my home to reap all these diverse health benefits.

Cold Plunge/Cold Water Exposure

When we stay immersed in iced water (50-60 degrees F), we intentionally trick our body into severe threat or stress (the process is called hormesis) that allows our body to improve the ability to adapt to adversity and, in turn, helps to promote resilience and boost mitochondrial functioning. Stay immersed in the cold plunge for at least one minute, ideally 2 to 3 minutes, to trigger the benefits. If access to cold plunge equipment is not available, we can alternatively immerse in a tub of ice-cold water or take a cold shower.

Lymphatic Drainage

We can improve lymphatic drainage on our own by sweating in a sauna, dry brushing, doing self-massage, foam rolling, walking, and doing yoga. We can also see a practitioner who specializes in lymphatic drainage massage. These practices help pump lymph fluid through the body, which helps with detoxification and immunity.

Not Smoking

Smoking directly damages mitochondrial quality and function because inhaling concentrated pollution directly into our bloodstream causes an extreme inflammatory response and oxidative stress. When quitting smoking, the body instantly goes to work on healing the damage that has been done. The sooner one quits smoking, the better.

Minimizing Alcohol Consumption

Drinking too much alcohol damages the liver, which is one of the most mitochondria-dense organs and is responsible for blood sugar metabolism. It is advisable to limit alcohol consumption to only one or two drinks per week or very occasionally for leisure or social situations.

Eating a Healthy Diet

A nutrient-rich, diverse diet provides our body with vitamins, minerals, and cofactors needed to produce energy. A phytonutrient-rich diet with adequate protein is the foundation for optimal metabolic processes in the body.

Exercise

When we exercise regularly, we send signals to our muscles to create more mitochondria and stem cells for overall vitality and peak potential. This especially works well when we exercise using a variety of protocols (HIIT, resistance training, weight training, cardio, yoga, and Pilates). Sweating through high-intensity interval training (HIIT) also helps to detoxify and lessen the burden of heavy metals on our body.

Maintaining a Healthy Body Weight

Obesity overloads and overwhelms the mitochondria, causing them to malfunction. This leads to inflammation and oxidative stress, which further damages mitochondria and accelerates aging. Therefore, maintaining a healthy body weight is essential for overall health.

Overview

In the right quantities, these supplements (micronutrients), as well as lifestyle practices, give our body the tools it needs to thrive on a cellular level. From a metabolic standpoint, they may help metabolize macronutrients, deliver energy to cells, regulate glucose, manage insulin production, reduce inflammation, and more. When we fall short of any of the primary macro and micronutrients, the body's natural metabolic processes can be disrupted, increasing our risk for poor health and a range of diseases and illnesses.

A Word of Caution

Once we know what vitamins and supplements we want to take, our next goal is to pick a high-quality, reputable brand. This is important because research shows that several low-quality supplements have been contaminated or adulterated with harmful bacteria, fungi, and heavy metals. Unlike prescription medication, the Food & Drug Administration (FDA) does not regulate vitamins and other supplements for safety and effectiveness before being marketed to the public.

To find a good supplement, look for brands that are third-party tested and stamped by the National Sanitation Foundation (NSF) International or U.S. Pharmacopeial Convention (USP) under the guidance and recommendation of a healthcare provider/expert.

CHAPTER 6

Optimal Diet - What, When, How to Eat

There is so much conflicting information available about "what to eat", that it's hard to know what is true. This chapter will guide us to understand how food matters. The food that you put into your body is not just for sustenance or calories; it is actually a crucial element of physical and mental health. Therefore, we should give it the time and respect it deserves by paying attention to what we eat, how we eat, and when we eat.

A "balanced diet" containing protein, healthy fats, vitamins, minerals, and other nutrients is needed for healthy tissue support, development, and protection. Fats and proteins are required to build and provide cells and tissue development, and vitamins and antioxidants, such as vitamins A, C, E, Zinc, and selenium, protect against free radicals and oxidative damage.

It is also important to consume a variety of food that supports digestive health. Without the proper breakdown of macronutrients (protein, fats, carbohydrates) and their absorption by the digestive system, our body can't provide the support needed for healthy tissues. And, of course, adequate hydration, sleep, and exercise are essential pieces to optimize cellular health, healing, repair, and detoxification. A balanced diet with the correct amount of calories is exactly what an individual's body needs to thrive. A plethora of trends and fad diets in food culture, availability, convenience, and an abundance of foods are leading people down a path of unhealthy eating that does the body more harm than good.

In my personal experience, food plays a huge role in my overall health journey. I found that mindful eating, following calorie restriction, paying attention to what, how, and when to eat, consuming probiotic and prebiotic-rich foods, eating enough protein, eating sufficient Omega-3 fatty acid-rich foods, and following the Mediterranean diet not only improved my overall well-being but helped me manage my autoimmune Hashimoto's thyroiditis. Over the past 5-7 years, I have had no symptoms of this condition, and that is without taking any immunosuppressive/immunomodulatory drugs.

Over the past several decades, our beneficial gut microbiome has taken a big hit due to the overuse and over-dependence of products that trigger autoimmune response:

- Antibiotics, antibacterial soap, hand sanitizers
- Harmful ingredients (parabens, phthalates) commonly present in skin care, fragrances, and hair care products
- Glyphosates, which are heavily present in insecticide and pesticide sprays on conventionally grown fruits and vegetables
- Grains, gluten, and glucose

Since gut bacteria have a direct impact on inflammation and immunity, hence damage to our gut microbiome makes us more susceptible to autoimmune disease. It is no surprise that autoimmunity and inflammation have been on a steep rise for the past several years. According to the American Autoimmune and Related Diseases Association (AARDA), approximately 50 million Americans (20% of the overall population) are suffering from an autoimmune disease (U.S. Department of Health and Human Services). But it is possible to manage autoimmunity by reducing the inflammation and healing the gut by feeding the microbiome the right nutrients, so the good bacteria sustain in the gut and optimize our digestive and immune health.

Aging, Disease, and Calorie Restriction

As we have already studied, aging is the slow accumulation of cellular damage and decreased ability to repair the damage. This results in a low level of inflammation called ***inflammaging*** that leads to chronic diseases and early death. Animal studies from as early as 1917 show that calorie restriction can prolong life, increase longevity, and prevent the development of cancer (McDonald, 2010; Flanagan, 2020). The concept is based on ***hormesis***, which is a phenomenon in which an intentionally low dose of stressors and biological damage strengthens and makes us more resistant to robust stressors. Calorie restriction is considered one of the hormesis that causes a rise in cortisol (stress hormone) and increases the production of heat shock proteins (HSP) that help to stabilize new proteins, repair the damaged ones, and hunker down inflammaging and oxidative stress (Selsby, 2005).

During our youth, we need to grow. However, during middle and older age, this high-growth program may cause premature aging. We know that the food we eat plays a large role in this growth cycle. Therefore, we need to make a deliberate adjustment to our diet to preserve our lifespan as well as our healthspan. Researchers have generally used a 40% calorie restriction guidance, but even a 10% calorie restriction in rats increased life by about 15%, whereas animals that were calorie-restricted by 40% lived 20% longer (Pifferi, 2018). Calorie restriction not only extends the lifespan but also slows and prevents age-related diseases, including dementia, diabetes, cardiovascular disease, neurodegenerative disorders, and several types of cancer (Flanagan, 2020).

One of the most compelling examples of calorie restriction in prolonging human lifespan can be found in Okinawa, Japan. Traditionally, Okinawans follow a practice of mindful eating by deliberately restricting when they are 80% full and effectively withholding 20% calorie restriction. This trend of a low-calorie diet (20% fewer calories) is indicative and supportive of the statistics that show 4-5 times more centenarians among their population than in most industrialized countries (Suzuki M. et al., 2001).

How Much We Should Eat

When our goal is weight loss, we should follow a **calorie-deprivation** diet, which is eating less than what our body burns per day. **Calorie restriction mode** is when we eat exactly what our body needs. This results in weight maintenance. If our goal is weight gain, then we should follow a **calorie-surplus diet**, which means eating more calories than we need.

Ideally, we should consume and split our meals as the breakdown below based on our overall goals:

- 30% Breakfast
- 30% Lunch
- 10% Snack
- 30% Dinner

I recommend maintaining a minimum 12-hour fasting window between dinner and breakfast—for example, finishing dinner by 7:00 PM and eating breakfast no earlier than 7:00 AM the following day. For example, intermittent fasting (IF), which means going without food for some time, has many benefits. It helps with anti-aging, helps our body manage insulin (Song, 2023), optimizes autophagy (Liu et al., 2023) (breaking down of senescent cells), and optimizes our nutrient-sensing pathways (DiFrancesco, 2018) (insulin and mTOR decreases while AMPK pathway increases).

Avoid extreme fasting and binge/cheat days, as they disrupt our body's natural balance. Extreme fasting can cause us to enter starvation mode, which causes our body to break down healthy tissue and disrupt our biochemistry.

Intermittent fasting disclaimer:

- If you are a young, healthy, fertile woman in your 20-30s, you don't need to do intermittent fasting as it might be detrimental to your fertility.

- If you have hormonal issues like polycystic ovarian syndrome (PCOS), endometriosis, hypothyroidism, or hyperthyroidism, then don't indulge in intermittent fasting without consulting your physician.

- If you are a young, healthy female athlete, you don't need to do intermittent fasting as you are already metabolically flexible; you are more likely to experience hormonal issues. In this case, your priority is to make sure that you eat right without limiting calories.

- If you are someone dealing with a lot of stress, then you should focus on recovery from stress rather than fasting.

Preventing Weight Gain and Obesity

Obesity contributes to Type 2 diabetes and other conditions that can shorten our lives. A healthy and lean body is associated with the lowest mortality rates in men and women of all ages (Lee, 2018). An ideal body mass index (BMI) of 20-24 is considered to be healthy; below 20 is underweight, above 25 is overweight, and greater than 30 is obese (Centers for Disease Control and Prevention, 2022). Overweight and obese people have more visceral fat, indicative of strong risk factors for diabetes.

You can calculate your BMI at https://www.aarp.org/health/healthy-living/info-2017/bmi_calculator.html.

Weight gain increases the risk of the following conditions:

- Coronary heart disease
- Type-2 diabetes
- Cancers (endometrial, breast, and colon)
- High blood pressure
- High total cholesterol
- High triglyceride level
- Sleep apnea and respiratory problems
- Osteoarthritis
- Infertility
- Stroke

A healthy diet helps to lose weight by:

- Lowering blood pressure
- Managing blood sugar
- Reducing LDL cholesterol level

Macronutrients

A balanced diet is composed of three important macronutrients - protein, fat, and carbohydrates. The ideal macronutrient ratio is:

- 25-30% fat
- 40% protein
- 30% carbohydrates

The ratio doesn't have to be perfect, but we want to maintain a healthy balance. While some food makes us feel better, many others can do the opposite. When we eat anything with sugar or flour, or more importantly, start the day by consuming sugar/excess carbs, especially if we do it on a daily basis or multiple times per day, our insulin level spikes, which causes fat storage and turns testosterone into estrogen, which can lead to weight gain and hormonal imbalance. We also age faster because fat accumulation leads to oxidative damage in the surrounding tissue, causing damage to DNA and cellular proteins. Thankfully, eating a whole-food diet rich in fiber, phytonutrients, and antioxidants helps to repair this damage and decelerates the speed of aging.

Not all fats are bad for us. Good fats, such as nuts, fish, coconut oil, omega-3 fatty acids (salmon, avocado, walnuts, and chia seeds), olive oil, macadamia nut oil, pumpkin seed oil, healthy meats like grass-fed beef and lamb, chicken and duck are highly beneficial for reducing inflammation, boosting immunity, strengthening the muscles and connective tissue, improving skin, brain and heart health.

Optimal Protein Intake

Protein is an essential macronutrient that is required as a building block to build and repair muscles, bones, hormones, and enzymes. Hence, it is important for growth, development, energy, and strength. Our optimal daily protein intake depends on our weight, age, goal, and level of physical activity. Eat enough protein from pasture-raised animals, eggs, wild-caught fish, and plant proteins. Consume an additional 30 grams of grass-fed collagen for connective tissue strength.

Daily intake of Protein:

- Sedentary - Aim for 1.2 - 1.8 grams/kg body weight
- Active, healthy, and wish to maintain a healthy weight - Aim for 1.4 - 2.0 grams/kg body weight
- Active, healthy, and want to build muscle - Aim for 1.6 - 2.4 grams/kg body weight
- Overweight - Aim for 1.2 - 1.5 grams/kg body weight
- Pregnant - Aim for 1.7 - 1.8 grams/kg body weight
- Seniors wishing to build muscle - Aim for 1.7 - 2.0 grams/kg body weight

As we age, the biggest threats to our lives are frailty, falls, and fractures due to decreased muscle strength and bone density. Sarcopenia is a muscle disorder defined as an impairment of physical function determined by walking speed and grip strength. Sarcopenia is the primary age-related cause of frailty. It is associated with a higher risk of disabilities in performing our daily tasks, and higher risk of having to go to nursing homes, higher risk of experiencing falls, fractures, and hospitalization (Papadopoulou, 2020). The older we get, the greater our muscles' anabolic resistance (i.e., their resistance to growth). Therefore, elderly people must eat more proteins to stimulate muscle protein synthesis to increase lean body mass and body composition.

The protein requirements stated so far were based on studies conducted on omnivores. ***People whose diet is mostly or entirely plant-based*** might need higher protein intake due to low-quality proteins, low bioavailability, and low amino acid profile. Essential amino acid (EAA) deficit of plant protein can be overcome by eating more protein, combining complementary proteins, and supplementing with **leucine** (Mariotti, 2019).

In general, for easy and simple protein-requirement calculations, every individual should aim for at least 100 grams of protein per day for overall health and wellness.

Micronutrients

Micronutrients are essential nutrients that the body requires in small amounts but play a crucial role in maintaining overall health and well-being. These include vitamins and minerals for various physiological functions.

Vitamins play a major role in growth, development, and metabolic processes. Vitamin A supports vision, immune function, and skin health. Vitamin C is a crucial antioxidant and supports collagen formation. Vitamin D is important for bone health, immune health, and mood regulation. Vitamin E is an antioxidant and an integral part of skin cells. Vitamin K is essential for blood clotting, bone health, and heart health.

Minerals are the substances that are crucial for various bodily functions, supporting bones, nerves, and enzymes. Some of the important minerals are calcium, iron, magnesium, Zinc, and selenium. Adequate intake of micronutrients is essential to support optimal health and aging.

Foods to Eat

A "balanced diet" containing protein, healthy fats (Omega-3 fatty acids), vitamins (A, C, D, E, K), minerals (Zinc, potassium, and selenium), and antioxidants (carotenoids and lycopene) is needed for healthy tissue support, development, and protection from oxidative damage.

What To Eat	What It Does
Red peppers, pumpkin, carrots, apricots, cantaloupe, sweet potatoes, broccoli, leafy greens	**Carotenoids** These highly pigmented foods are rich in vitamin A and boost skin health and glow
Tomatoes, watermelon, red peppers, pink grapefruit	**Lycopene** Helps cellular repair and renewal Boosts skin's natural SPF
Bananas, beet greens, Swiss chard, sweet potatoes, avocados, cooked lentils	**Potassium** Essential mineral for neutralizing toxins and acidity. Vital for heart health, bone health, muscle function and electrolyte balance
Sweet potatoes and yams, carrots, butternut squash, kale, spinach	**Vitamin A** Boosts eye health since everyone's eyesight starts to diminish after the age of 40 Skin looks young and vibrant, creating a healthy glow
Lamb (provides 100% of daily requirement of B2), almonds, avocados, beets, mushrooms	**Vitamin B2 (Riboflavin)** Boosts metabolism Reduces inflammation Maintains eye health

Almonds, sweet potatoes, egg yolks, avocado	**Vitamin B7 (Biotin)** Supports healthy hair and strong nails
Garbanzo beans, lentils, pinto beans, asparagus	**Vitamin B9 (Folate)** Crucial for proper cell division and growth, red blood cell formation, and plays a major role in the production of neurotransmitters like serotonin, dopamine, and norepinephrine.
Oranges, grapefruit, kiwis, spinach, red and green peppers, Brussels sprouts, cantaloupe	**Vitamin C** Increases collagen production, excellent for skin health
Sunflower seeds, almonds, hazelnuts, spinach, asparagus, avocado	**Vitamin E** It is an anti-aging powerhouse that maintains youthfulness, elasticity, and hydration of skin cells. It is a great source of antioxidants that protect against free radicals, oxidative damage, and inflammation. It also supports healthy immune function.
Spinach, dandelion greens, kale, broccoli, Brussels sprouts	**Vitamin K** It boosts bone density, helps with blood clotting, and strengthens blood vessels.
Lentils, pumpkin seeds, kidney beans	**Zinc (Zn)** It's an essential mineral that supports the immune system and prevents infection. Due to its anti-inflammatory properties, Zn helps in collagen production and reduces acne and

	other inflammatory skin conditions like eczema, psoriasis, and rashes.
	Boosts cognitive function and reduces the risk of age-related cognitive decline.

Foods to Avoid

While some foods make us feel and look better, many others do just the opposite. When we eat food with sugar or grains on a daily basis or multiple times per day, the following tends to happen:

- Our insulin spikes, which metabolically results in fat storage.

- Our testosterone spikes, which then gets converted to estrogen, leading to weight gain and hormonal imbalance, which is a major cause of the trending exponential increase in pre-menstrual syndrome (PMS), fibroids, and endometriosis in women.

- The rate of aging is accelerated because inflammation-inducing foods cause oxidation, DNA and cellular protein damage, exacerbating cellular death.

Thankfully, eating whole foods optimizes the aging process by fueling our body to make its own antioxidants.

What Not To Eat	What It Does
Margarine, chips, crackers, fast food, baked goods	**Trans fat (hydrogenated oil)**
	Inflammation, diabetes, heart attacks, heart disease, and stroke (Pipoyan, 2021)

Bread, candy, flavored yogurt, salad dressings, cereals, and most shelf-stable processed foods	**High Fructose Corn Syrup/Sugar** Most of these processed foods have preservatives, high fructose, emulsifiers, dyes, and chemicals that are highly toxic to the body and disrupt our hormones and fatty acid metabolism. White sugar or high fructose corn syrup wreaks havoc on our body, is highly addictive, and causes steep blood sugar rise and crash, which has been linked to a range of diseases, including cancer, diabetes, and obesity. It also damages our gut, collagen, and elastin, causing rapid skin aging.
"Sugar-free" foods, diet soda, desserts, sugar-free gum, baked goods, drink mixes, cereal, breath mints, toothpaste and some chewable vitamins	**Artificial Sweeteners (Sucralose, aspartame, saccharin)** Increased risk of Alzheimer's, Parkinson's, fibromyalgia, diabetes, lymphoma, brain tumors, multiple sclerosis, chronic fatigue, mental and emotional disorders (depression, anxiety attacks, mental confusion, etc.), seizures, migraines, and cancer (Czarnecka. 2021)
Candy, drinks, cereal, cheese, baked goods, ice cream	**Artificial Colors (Red 40, Yellow 5 and 6, Blue 1 and 2)** These dyes have been linked to ADHD, thyroid cancer, and chromosomal damage (Potera, 2010).

Bacon, ham, hot dogs, lunch meat, cured meat, corned beef, smoked fish, and other processed meats	**Sodium Nitrites & Nitrates** Damage to internal organs, particularly liver and pancreas Linked to increased risk of breast and prostate cancer (Chazelas, 2022)
Chinese food, snack foods, seasonings, soup products, frozen dinners, and lunch meats	**MSG (Monosodium Glutamate)** Flavor enhancer that is commonly used in processed foods, restaurant meats, and packaged snacks has been associated with various forms of toxicity (neurotoxicity) and linked with increased risk of obesity and metabolic disorders (Olney, 1994). Linked to neurological issues such as depression, disorientation, fatigue, headaches, eye damage, and obesity (Niaz, 2018).
Potato chips, gum, cereal, frozen sausage, vegetable oils, enriched rice, candy, lard, shortening, and Jell-O	**Butylated Hydroxyanisole (BHA) and Butylated Hydroxytoluene (BHT)** Endocrine disruptor and causes cancer-causing reactive compounds to form in the body, resulting in potential risk for cancers.
Non-organic dairy and meat	**Antibiotics & Growth Hormones** It induces dysbiosis, an imbalance between good and bad bacteria in the gut that can lead to yeast infections, candida, and leaky gut syndrome. Increased risk of obesity and some forms of cancer (Jeong, 2010).

Be Mindful of Hydration

> *"Drinking water should be so natural that you don't even think about it."*

On average, the body loses 2-3 quarts of water per day. Suboptimal hydration may raise the stress hormone Cortisol, which causes metabolism to slow down, creating a resistance to weight loss. These fluids need to be replaced for optimal body function; **"hydration is essential."**

The best source of hydration is water, which is a game changer for our body, brain, and beauty. Our skin looks plumper and fresher when we're hydrated. Water also flushes out toxins, which improves and optimizes health and aging.

Every morning, I like to add lemon juice to my glass of water to cleanse, alkalize, and boost immunity. It is also a good practice to add a pinch of Celtic salt to water since it is a healthier option to table salt due to its mineral richness and less-processed nature. It ramps up the hydration by enhancing the osmolarity of the cells.

Ideally, women should drink 11.5 cups (2.7 liters), and men should drink 15.5 cups (3.7 liters) of water per day, according to the U.S. National Academies of Sciences, Engineering, and Medicine (U.S. National Academies of Sciences, Engineering, and Medicine, 2004).

One simple way to calculate our daily water intake in ounces is to aim for half our body weight in pounds each day to stay well hydrated. Building a habit of sipping water intermittently and regularly is more beneficial than chugging it all at once. We should slow down our consumption later in the day, as downing glass after glass, especially toward the end of the day, can lead to overhydration and waking up throughout the night.

Alcohol

Drinking too much alcohol damages the liver, disrupts blood sugar metabolism, and depletes vitamins, minerals, and fluids out of the body. It's advisable to limit your alcohol to 1-2 drinks/week or very occasionally. Spirits like tequila, vodka, and scotch (served on the rocks or with club soda) are a better choice than wine because of their lower sugar content. To avoid a hangover the day after a night out, a little trick is to consume plenty of hydrating fluids like coconut water (8 oz.), B-complex vitamins, foods rich in vitamin C, and bone broth with ginger.

We now have all of the tools that we need to determine how to correct food intake in moderation and balance but also an extensive list of what to avoid and what to eat to slow the aging process and age-related diseases.

CHAPTER 7

Sleep Is the Key to Longevity

Everything that has life sleeps one way or another: dolphins, birds, fish, bacteria, and even viruses. This is what indicates how important sleep is. Roughly one third of our lives is spent sleeping because it is that important for health.

I would argue that sleep is the single most effective thing that we can do to reset our brain, body, and health. If we were to compare the factors like exercise, food, and water versus a lack of sleep for 24 hours and then map our brain and body impairments, we would notice that one night of lost sleep has a more harmful impact on our body than the other factors.

According to data reported in Garner, 2019, 79% of the US population sleeps less than 8 hours, 70% of the UK population and 90% of the Japanese population reported less than 8 hours of sleep, supporting the notion that millions of people struggle with insufficient sleep, emphasizing a global epidemic of sleep deprivation.

We have this belief in our society that less sleep equals more productivity. However, this couldn't be further from the truth. Insufficient sleep costs the United States about $411 billion annually, with Japan facing a staggering $138 billion in economic losses (Hafner, 2016). A lack of sleep not only causes employees to miss work, but it increases rate of obesity and risk of cardiovascular disease and mental health.

Benefits of sufficient sleep

The list of benefits of sleep is endless. We know that sleep boosts our immune system, regulates our blood sugar levels, controls our appetite hormones (leptin and ghrelin) and metabolism, regulates the sex hormones (testosterone and estrogen), improves memory, helps maintain muscle mass, and helps us learn and remember. Sleep de-escalates anxiety, reduces emotional difficulties and traumas, and helps cleanse away Alzheimer's toxic proteins (beta-amyloid) that build up in the brain. Patterns of insufficient sleep have been linked to greater insulin resistance, metabolic abnormalities, and weight gain, which might then result in diabetes and adverse cardiovascular outcomes (Liu, 2016).

Health implications of sleep deprivation

When people sleep for less than 6-7 hours per night, they become more vulnerable to a whole host of serious health problems. There is not one major organ within the body or the process within the brain that isn't affected by sleep.

Let's look at some of these.

1. Short-term – When we are deprived of sleep, we start to have what we call microsleeps, where our eyelids will partially close unintentionally and our brain seems to be falling asleep. This microsleep can last for 1-2 seconds, which is detrimental enough for us to drift from one lane to the next while driving.

2. Mid-term – A consistent lack of sleep creates a cascade of health problems. Initially, it triggers pre-diabetes, reduced sex hormone production, and elevated blood pressure. These changes accelerate the development of serious conditions, including obesity, diabetes, and cardiovascular disease. Mental health deteriorates as well, with increased rates of anxiety and depression. Cognitive abilities suffer too—decision-making, creativity, planning, memory, and communication all become impaired, while persistent brain fog becomes the new normal. Emotions get impacted, causing mood swings, stress, depression, and angry outbursts due to sleeplessness and related fatigue. Sleeping less than 6-7 hours per night diminishes our immune system. Studies in which patients have been deprived of sleep for one week have shown an increased risk of immune-compromised infection (Garbarino, 2021).

3. Long-term – The shorter we sleep, the shorter our life span. Insufficient sleep increases the risk of all-cause mortality by 12% (Cappuccio, 2010).

Researchers have discovered that a history of insufficient sleep could increase the risk of dementia by 20% (Goldman, 2023). People who, on average, sleep six hours or less have a far higher magnitude of beta-amyloid protein related to Alzheimer's disease. We also know that two sleep disorders, insomnia and sleep apnea (heavy snoring), are associated with a marked increased risk of Alzheimer's disease later in life (Brzecka,

2018). We now have the causal evidence in animal models and human models indicating if a human being is deprived of sleep for a single night, there is an immediate increase in these Alzheimer's disease-related proteins circulating in the brain.

During deep sleep, the brain's glymphatic system (waste clearance mechanism) becomes highly active. This system functions like a powerful cleansing process that flushes away harmful metabolic byproducts, particularly beta-amyloid and tau proteins—the two primary molecules associated with Alzheimer's disease development (Michaud, 2023). Without sufficient deep sleep, these toxins accumulate, potentially accelerating cognitive decline.

It may not be a coincidence that Margaret Thatcher and Ronald Reagan, both known for being short sleepers, went on to die of the unfortunate disease of Alzheimer's.

Therefore, it is very important to self-check for the signs of sleep deprivation by keeping a close watch on three sleep patterns noticed recurrently, which are sleep duration of less than 4-5 hours per night, frequent urge for daytime naps, and taking more than thirty minutes to fall asleep (aka latency period).

Different Stages of Sleep

During sleep, the brain is extremely active. In fact, the brain actually goes through different sleep stages, each performing various functions:

1. Non-rapid eye movement (1): This stage is where we transition from being awake to sleeping and typically

lasts only 5-10 minutes and is often shallow sleep. During this period, as the body relaxes, some people might even say, "I wasn't sleeping" during this stage when woken.

2. Non-rapid eye movement (2): The body slows down and falls into a pattern of regular breathing and heart rate. Brain waves are functioning to consolidate and filter memories acquired throughout the day.

3. Non-rapid eye movement (3): This stage, also known as delta or deep sleep, typically occurs early in the sleep cycle when the muscles are relaxed and breathing slows. When we are in delta sleep, we are not easily woken up by noises around us.

4. Rapid eye movement sleep (REM) or dream sleep: REM sleep typically begins 90 minutes after falling asleep and serves to consolidate memories, and process and store emotions. It is also an important stage for learning.

Factors that Impact Sleep

There are many factors that can inhibit not only the quantity but the quality of sleep we get each night.

Caffeine and Sleep

Caffeine affects our sleep in several ways. When we're awake during the day, we build up a sleepiness chemical in our brains called adenosine. The longer we're awake, the more adenosine builds up, making us sleepy toward the end of the day. When we sleep, the brain clears away all of that adenosine during a full night of 7-9 hours of sleep to feel refreshed and restored the next day.

1. Caffeine is a stimulant that makes us more alert and more awake. But how does it work? It is no coincidence that caffeine and adenosine sound the same at the end; caffeine forces away the adenosine and hijacks those receptors. By latching on adenosine receptors, caffeine prevents adenosine molecules from binding to these sites, thereby blocking the signal that would normally cause drowsiness. This is why caffeine is often used to stay awake and alert. Even though we may not feel sleepy anymore after caffeine consumption, adenosine is still there and, in fact, continues to build, leading to what we call the caffeine crash.

2. Duration of action: Caffeine has a half-life of about six hours. Therefore, the last cup of coffee should not be later than 2 pm.

3. Caffeine blocks deep sleep and strips it away by 15 to 30 percent. We know by now how critical deep sleep is. It's the time when we replenish our immune system and regulate our metabolic system, which controls the hormones such as insulin that regulate our blood sugar. Deep sleep also strengthens, consolidates, and secures new memories in our brains, preventing those memories from being forgotten.

> Deep sleep is also the time when the brain's waste removal system operates most efficiently, a critical process for long-term brain health that we discussed earlier in relation to Alzheimer's risk.

The data associated with coffee and its health benefits is immensely compelling. Study after study makes it strikingly clear that drinking coffee is good for our overall health. In studies about decaffeinated coffee, the results are very similar about the health benefits, indicating that it's not the caffeine but the coffee itself. So the bottom line here is to drink coffee, but I would say the dose and the timing are critical, so try to limit ourselves to about two cups of coffee per day to maximize the health benefits, as more than that might cause more harm than good.

Blue Light

With artificial lighting around us all day, it is understandable that the blue light emitted from devices would impact our brains and, more importantly, our sleep in some way. In a study conducted by Harvard Medical School, it was shown that reading for an hour on an iPad just before bed versus reading a book in dim light affects the latency period (time to fall asleep) as well as the total duration of sleep. Lastly, blue light from these devices delays the release of the hormone melatonin by 90 minutes to 2 hours, affecting our brain to think it is still daytime (Harvard Health, 2020).

Insufficient sleep not only makes us want to eat more but also to crave heavy-hitting starchy foods like bread, pasta, and pizza. This is due to appetite-regulating hormones, leptin, and ghrelin, getting imbalanced due to insufficient sleep. For example, leptin tells us when we are satiated and no longer need to consume more food. Ghrelin, on the other hand, does the opposite; it says we're not satisfied, and we still want to eat more. In some of the first sleep studies, scientists started to restrict people's sleep to just 4-5 hours and what they found was that overall hunger levels rose by about 26 percent (Cooper, 2018). In other words, on average, underslept individuals started to eat 300-400 extra calories.

Studies have found that when we are sleep deprived, naturally occurring endocannabinoids in our body (control appetite) skyrocket by over 20%, cranking up people's appetite (Easton, 2016). Endocannabinoids increase our preference for simple sugars and cravings for salty foods, hence increasing blood pressure and affecting cardiovascular health. "If the name sounds familiar, that's because this hormone acts in the same way that Cannabis does when smoked or taken as an edible, causing people to become viciously hungry."

Hormonal issues/Obesity/Timing of meals/Exercise

Our bodies are built to burn fat at night as we sleep to lose excess weight. Sleep deprivation is associated with growth hormone deficiency and elevated cortisol levels, both of which have been linked to obesity (Sleep Foundation.org, 2023). The effect of sleep loss on weight is not limited to only hormones, but restricted sleep duration has been shown to cause a greater tendency to select high-calorie food (Greer et al., 2013). Calories consumed late at night increase the risk of weight gain. Furthermore, adults who do not get sufficient sleep get less exercise than those who do, possibly because of sleepiness and fatigue during the day (Kline CE, 2014).

Alcohol

Some people use alcohol as a sleep aid, but in fact, alcohol leads to a night of poor, restless, and fragmented sleep because alcohol has negative effects on REM sleep, which is probably the most restorative sleep. Therefore, we wake up in the morning not feeling refreshed and rested.

Drinking alcohol before bed can also worsen sleep apnea, where the airways collapse and block during sleep because alcohol is a muscle relaxer, and it can slack airway muscles, causing them to obstruct waking us up, choking and gasping for air.

Key Things to Do

To improve our chances of healthy, deep sleep to optimize your health and performance, follow these standard tips for improved "sleep hygiene."

1. Insomnia: If we have insomnia, don't nap during the day. Even if we don't struggle with sleep at night, we should try not to nap late in the afternoon or early evening. But if we don't struggle with sleep, naps are

wonderful things. Just keep in mind the 20-minute limit for a nap.

2. Sleep schedule: We should aim to go to bed at the same time and wake up at the same time during the weekday or the weekend because our brain expects and thrives amidst regularity. In order to do things effectively during the day, we need cortisol, adrenaline, and noradrenaline. But if we miss our ideal sleep window, the body's circadian rhythm gets messed up and these critical hormones and neurostimulants can lead to insomnia. That is why going to bed at the right and consistent time is critical since we are designed for regularity as Dr. Walker explains, "If you feed your brain regularity, which is what it wishes for and expects, the quantity and quality of sleep will improve" (Walker, 2019).

3. Sleep environment (Darkness/temperature): With all of the distractions, devices, and light, we do not experience enough darkness to signal to our brain that it is time for sleep. 1-2 hours before our scheduled bedtime, we should dim or turn off all lights in the house. We should aim for a bedroom temperature of about 18.5 degrees Celsius or around 65 to 68 degrees Fahrenheit. We need to reduce our core body and brain temperature by about one degree Celsius to fall asleep and stay asleep. If we find ourselves lying awake for 30 minutes or more, get up

and walk out or do something different, but don't lie in bed awake for longer.

4. Electronics: Avoid electronics at night and consider installing blackout curtains in our bedroom because turning down the lights surrounding us triggers the release of melatonin that helps to regulate sleep.

5. Sunlight: Expose ourselves to sunlight first thing when we wake up to kickstart our circadian rhythm.

6. Meal Timing: Stop eating 4-6 hours before bedtime because the carbs and proteins we eat within four hours of sleep will inhibit our prolactin surge and spike our insulin. We know prolactin is an important hormone in regulating sleep. Prolactin levels naturally peak, particularly during REM sleep, and has been associated with promoting deep sleep and overall improved sleep quality.

7. Alcohol: When going out, it's best to limit alcohol to a moderate amount which is generally defined as up to 2 drinks per night for men and 1 drink per night for women. The key is to drink in moderation and allow enough time for the body to metabolize the alcohol before bedtime. It is recommended to stop drinking at least 4 hours before bed to prevent sleep disruption.

8. Caffeine: Try to limit caffeine consumption to 2 cups of coffee per day because of its health benefits

but the last cup of coffee should not be later than 2 pm.

9. Sleep aid supplements: Consider supplements like magnesium, L-Theanine, lavender oil, and ashwagandha that relax and calm our mind and see how our body responds.

10. Sleep trackers: Sleep trackers are a good place to start. What gets measured gets managed. One of the most popular wearable devices for tracking sleep is the Oura Ring, which delivers overall sleep scores and detailed analysis of different stages of sleep (deep, REM sleep), restlessness of the previous night, readiness for the next day, and heart rate variability (HRV). It is like a dream come true for biohackers, athletes, and health-conscious individuals eager to better understand their sleep data. Many of Oura Ring users have reported improved sleep and better quality of life after making simple changes to their lifestyle and sleep hygiene, such as maintaining a consistent bedtime, avoiding late-night eating or drinking, and limiting exposure to electronics or blue light in the bedroom.

11. If sleep deprivation seems extreme, we should consult a doctor for serious sleep disorders like severe insomnia or obstructive sleep apnea, a condition in which our breathing is repeatedly interrupted. On a personal level, aim to follow a lifestyle that supports healthy weight and blood pressure and avoid smoking.

12. Audio-Visual Stimulation: One of my favorite biohacks is using brainTap's audio-visual stimulation technology, which helps activate the brain's peak potential and engage different neural pathways for a more balanced and focused state of mind. This technique combines sound and light therapy, where flashing lights at specific frequencies are delivered to the eyes and ears. These frequencies signal the nervous system to shift out of fight or flight mode and enter into state of relaxation. This process releases the neurotransmitter "GABA" that is an inhibitory neurotransmitter that helps to calm, promote relaxation and reduce anxiety and induce sleep.

CHAPTER 8

Measure Yourself - If You Don't Measure, You Can't Manage

One of the most valuable tools in diagnostics is the variety of blood tests/biomarkers to have an ongoing snapshot of your health and to help your physician evaluate if your body is operating within the right parameters. These biomarkers analyze everything from nutrient levels (minerals, vitamins, and omega-3 fatty acids), insulin and glucose markers, cholesterol, inflammatory markers, hormone levels, and heavy metal testing. It is important that we monitor our health for any alarming changes that we notice in our lab investigation to ensure our health and well-being.

What are biomarkers? Biomarkers are indicators of our body's physiological state. These markers are measured by analyzing blood and urine samples. Biomarkers tell us about the current state of our body as they change based on improving diet, lifestyle, and state of health. This range of modern-day biomarker testing is available through companies like Quest Diagnostics and LabCorp.

Routine Lab Tests to Detect the Root Cause of Disease

To be proactive in diagnosis and prevention, the following basic and advanced tests need to be routinely conducted and followed up with your physician.

Basic Testing

1. Heart health: Heart health refers to the health of our cardiovascular system, including arteries, vessels, and more. Blood biomarkers of heart health can also indicate our body's ability to transport and clear cholesterol from the body.

   Key markers of heart health include ApoB, HDL cholesterol, and resting heart rate.

   The risk factors for heart disease include high blood pressure, high low-density lipoprotein (LDL) cholesterol, diabetes, smoking and secondhand smoke exposure, obesity, unhealthy diet, physical inactivity (Centers for Disease Control and Prevention, 2022), and a family history of heart disease.

   - Total cholesterol: Less than 200 mg/dL is desirable, 200–239 mg/dL is considered borderline, and 240 mg/dL and above is high.

   - LDL cholesterol: LDL has traditionally been referred to as "bad" cholesterol for its reported role in heart disease risk. When LDL levels are high for long periods, accompanied by inflammation, that increases the risk of plaque formation in the blood vessels. Measurements under 130 mg/dL are generally acceptable.

   - ApoB testing: This measurement determines the amount of a protein, ApoB, which assists in clearing cholesterol from the blood and is prominent in LDL cholesterol. Levels over 110 mg/dL may indicate a higher risk of heart disease.

- LDL particle testing: This blood test measures the number and size of the LDL particles in our blood. An increase of small, dense LDL particles may indicate a greater risk of heart disease and insulin resistance.

- HDL cholesterol: HDL cholesterol is typically identified as "good" cholesterol as it removes excess cholesterol from the bloodstream, carrying it back to the liver to be broken down and eliminated. Optimal HDL cholesterol levels indicate a healthy heart. Ideally, 60 mg/dL or higher is desired, and levels below 40 mg/dL increase the risk of heart disease (Schaefer, 2010).

- Triglycerides: Triglycerides are a type of fat found in the blood. High triglyceride levels–typically above 150 mg/dL–are associated with an increased risk of cardiovascular disease.

2. Metabolism: Our body's metabolism reflects the processes in the body that consume and use energy for the growth, repair, and maintenance of cells, tissues, and organs. Our metabolic biomarkers reflect the efficiency of this process.

Key markers of metabolic health include glucose, HbA1c, insulin, thyroid hormones (T3, T4), and thyroid-stimulating hormone (TSH).

Blood glucose levels and insulin levels are essential indicators of our overall metabolic health, also serving as a warning sign of potential metabolic dysfunction. Standard testing for diabetes includes fasting glucose and hemoglobin A1c and fasting insulin.

- Fasting glucose test: A level of 70 to 99 mg/dL (3.9 and 5.5 mmol/L) is considered normal (Blood Sugar Test, 2024)

- Hemoglobin A1c (HbA1c): HbA1c represents the average amount of glucose in your blood for the past 90-120 days. Glucose can bind to the hemoglobin inside the red blood cells, if not used quickly. Optimal HbA1c of less than 5.5% is associated with increased longevity (Sikaris, 2009).

- Fasting insulin test: Elevated fasting insulin and glucose levels can signal that the body is becoming insulin resistant, indicating the early progression towards pre-diabetes. This condition warrants both lifestyle and medical intervention such as continuous glucose monitoring to prevent further decline. Maintaining insulin levels between 2.5 and 18.4 micro-IU/mL is generally recommended. This marker is especially critical because an estimated 1 in 3 Americans has pre-diabetes, 1 in 10 has Type 2 diabetes, and nearly 20% of individuals with diabetes remain undiagnosed.

- Thyroid-stimulating hormone (TSH): TSH is the most sensitive marker of thyroid health. It's released from the pituitary gland in the brain and acts on the thyroid gland and its hormones, triiodothyronine (T3) and thyroxine (T4). Thyroid hormones are closely tied to metabolic processes, body temperature regulation, and nervous system development.

3. Micronutrient testing: Micronutrient testing is extremely critical for detecting the physiological functioning of cells.

    Key markers of micronutrients include Ferritin, Vitamin B12, Zinc, Copper, Vitamin D, and Calcium.

    - Ferritin indicates the amount of iron stored in the body: The normal range is 24 to 336 micrograms per liter for men and 11 to 307 micrograms per liter for women.

    - Vitamin B12 plays an essential role in producing red blood cells, converting food into energy, and creating DNA in the body. Measurements below 400 pg/mL are considered low and require supplemental B12.

    - Zinc and copper: Zinc helps our body create protein and keeps our immune system running, while copper helps make energy, connective tissue, and blood vessels. Women should have zinc levels over 70 mcg/dL and copper levels higher than 80 mcg/dL. For men, zinc should be more than 74 mcg/dL, and copper should be higher than 70 mcg/dL (US Department of Health and Human Services, 2022).

- Vitamin D: Vitamin D helps our body absorb calcium and phosphorus to build and maintain bone health. The correct dosage depends on our blood levels of vitamin D in ng/ml. If blood levels are below 30 ng/ml, a threshold considered insufficient, it is generally recommended to supplement with 1000 IU per day of vitamin D daily (according to the National Institutes of Health) but no more than 2000 IU. (US Department of Health and Human Services, 2023). Vitamin D also promotes sleep quality, improves athletic performance, and supports overall longevity.

- Calcium: Optimal calcium levels and intake from the diet are critical to lowering the risk of osteoporosis and stress fractures.

4. Cognition: Cognition reflects the body's brain and nerve function, impacting reaction time and mood. Cognitive biomarkers indicate our ability to focus, process information, and consolidate memories.

Key markers of cognition include cortisol, vitamin B12, and insulin.

Cortisol: The body releases cortisol in response to physical and emotional stress. It helps regulate energy, metabolism, and immune function. Chronically high cortisol levels are associated with poor sleep quality, impaired blood sugar control, increased anxiety, depressed moods, digestive problems, and loss of muscle mass.

5. Sleep: Sleep is paramount for the body's repair processes and memory consolidation. Blood biomarker levels that can impact and are impacted by our ability to fall asleep and achieve good quality sleep are magnesium, vitamin D, glucose levels, as well as amount of deep sleep, and REM sleep.

6. Hormone balance: As we get older, our hormone levels begin to fluctuate and decrease between the ages of 40 and 50. This matters because hormones are the primary driver of energy, vitality, strength, power, focus, and beauty.

   Sex hormones not only govern sexual health but also play a vital role in physiologic functions such as blood sugar regulation, hormone regulation, cardiac and muscle health, bone metabolism, and brain health. It is important to detect hormonal deficiencies in order to supplement hormones to optimal levels for life-changing outcomes for men and women both.

   Key markers of hormone balance for men include total testosterone, free testosterone, dihydrotestosterone (DHT), sex hormone binding globulin (SHBG), dehydroepiandrosterone (DHEA), and cortisol.

   Key markers of hormone balance for women include estradiol (E2), progesterone, testosterone, SHBG, DHEA, and cortisol.

7. Recovery from exercise and stress: Recovery biomarkers provide insight into the body's response to exercise or physical activity across different intensities and durations.

Key markers of recovery include ALT, AST, creatine kinase, and magnesium.

- Alanine Aminotransferase (ALT): ALT is an enzyme found primarily in the liver. It is also found in other tissues, like the skeletal muscle. Elevated ALT levels in the blood may indicate liver or muscle cell damage.

- Magnesium: Magnesium supports healthy blood pressure and the immune system and assists in muscle contraction and relaxation. RBC magnesium levels are considered a more sensitive measure of magnesium as compared to serum magnesium.

- Aspartate aminotransferase (AST): AST is an enzyme found in the liver, heart, muscle tissue, and kidneys. This enzyme helps to metabolize proteins. High levels of AST in the blood likely indicate damage to tissues.

- Creatine kinase (CK): CK is found in muscle cells and plays a major role in producing energy during the first few seconds of exercise. Strenuous exercise can damage muscle cells, causing CK to leak into the blood. Optimal CK levels indicate that your muscle tissue is healthy.

8. Endurance: The endurance capacity indicates your ability to sustain cardiovascular and muscular activities. Endurance biomarkers reflect aerobic capacity, energy utilization, oxygen transport, and stamina.

Key markers of endurance include ferritin, hemoglobin, and vitamin B12.

9. Inflammation: Inflammation describes our body's ability to protect and respond to foreign substances, including pathogens, infections, viruses, and lifestyle stressors such as too much or too little exercise and sleep. Inflammation has been known to increase the risk of chronic health conditions such as heart disease or certain cancers.

    Key markers of inflammation include hs-CRP, ESR, homocysteine, and white blood cell count.

    Testing for undetected inflammation includes:

    - High-sensitivity C-reactive protein (hs-CRP) test: Hs-CRP can be used to diagnose long-term inflammatory conditions, such as heart disease, rheumatoid arthritis, lupus, or signs of infection.

    - Homocysteine: This amino acid is used in the body to make protein and to help diagnose inflammation. A normal level is 5–15 mmol/L.

    - ESR if elevated, indicate low levels of inflammation in the body.

10. Heavy metal toxicity: The Total Tox Bundle is a comprehensive test panel designed to assess heavy metal toxicity in the body. This bundle typically includes a combination of tests that measure the levels of various heavy metals in the blood, urine, or hair.

Some common heavy metals that are tested in the Total Tox Bundle include:

- Lead
- Mercury
- Cadmium
- Arsenic
- Aluminum
- Nickel
- Chromium

Heavy metal toxicity can occur due to exposure to environmental pollutants, contaminated food or water, gasoline, pesticides, and other metabolites through cosmetics and skincare. These are the worst offenders that impact our health much more than we actually realize.

Symptoms of heavy metal toxicity may vary depending on the type and level of exposure but can include fatigue, headaches, cognitive problems, digestive issues, increased risk of cancer, autism, asthma, allergies, infertility, obesity, and mitochondrial dysfunction, and cause more severe health effects if left untreated.

The Total Tox Bundle can provide valuable information about the levels of heavy metals in the body and help healthcare providers diagnose and treat heavy metal toxicity. If you suspect heavy metal toxicity or have concerns about exposure to heavy metals, it is recommended to consult with a healthcare provider for further evaluation and detox plans.

Advanced Testing

While blood and urine tests form the foundation of biomarker monitoring, several advanced technologies now allow us to look deeper into our health status and aging processes. These specialized assessments provide additional dimensions of health data that can further personalize your longevity strategy:

1. Bone Density DEXA Scan (Dual X-ray absorptiometry): Bone density is critical for long-term health. One in two women over the age of 50 suffer a fracture due to compromised bone density and bone strength. This test takes just 3 minutes with minimal radiation involved. I have personally done this test once a year for the past decade to scan and measure for osteoporosis.

2. DNA analysis: A comprehensive DNA analysis, including full genome sequencing, can provide valuable insights into our genetic risks for various health conditions. It can also help to predict how we might respond to certain medications and identify potential food intolerances. Understating our genetic predisposition such as higher or lower risk for certain cancers, can empower and guide us in making better lifestyle and healthcare decisions.

3. Microbiome analysis: It is an innovative clinical tool that measures gastrointestinal (GI) microbiome and its DNA from a single stool sample. This analysis can

help identify imbalances in the GI system that may contribute to digestive issues, poor gut health, or low energy levels.

4. Skin analysis: AI facial imaging analysis uses artificial intelligence to evaluate the health and age of our skin to identify sun damage and collagen depletion so doctors can customize an anti-aging plan to treat and prevent future skin damage.

5. Biological age testing: Some of us age faster than our chronological age and some slower. The simple epigenetic testing of our DNA determines our true biological age, including markers like telomere length and the pace of aging. This test is called TruAge. There is also another test known as GlycanAge, which estimates biological age by assessing the state of our immune system. I took the GlycanAge test last year at the chronological age of 51, and to my surprise, my biological age came back as just 30. That was incredibly encouraging and reaffirmed the impact of my lifestyle choices.

CHAPTER 9

Skin Health and Beauty – Unlocking the Radiance Within

When it comes to beauty, I am a firm believer that beauty starts from the inside out. It's just simple. Your health shows on your face. If you take care of yourself by eating the healthiest food possible, drinking sufficient water for hydration, and moving your body every day, then it shows on your face; you look and feel good and be comfortable and confident in your own skin.

But I also know that life happens and there will be times of stress due to travel, late nights, hormonal fluctuations (adolescence, pregnancy, and the transitions of menopause), and many other inevitable aspects in life. These shifts can affect our skin significantly. Thus, understanding how to adapt our skincare and makeup routines accordingly can be a game-changer, acting as a confidence booster during challenging times.

In this chapter, I aim to share my approach to beauty, which has always been centered on achieving healthy skin and a natural glow. It is essential to recognize that everyone's journey to health, wellness, and beauty is unique. That diversity is what inspired me to write this chapter. I hope to offer inspiration and practical tips on skin health that will empower you to become the best version of yourself.

This fundamental principle shapes my approach to skincare and wellness. When we prioritize our well-being, it not only enhances our appearance but also elevates our mood and boosts our confidence.

The Foundation: Inner Well-Being

Beauty begins with nurturing our inner selves. To cultivate radiant skin, we must first focus on what we consume. A diet filled with nutrient-dense foods rich in vitamins, minerals, and antioxidants provides the foundation for healthy skin. Eating whole foods, such as fruits, vegetables, nuts, and lean proteins, supports skin regeneration and repair. For instance, foods rich in Vitamin C, like oranges and bell peppers, can help promote collagen production, while omega-3 fatty acids found in fish can offer anti-inflammatory benefits.

Hydration is another cornerstone of skin health. Drinking plenty of water not only helps flush out toxins but also keeps our skin plump and youthful. The general guideline of 8 glasses of water (8 oz. each) per day can serve as a starting point, but always adjust according to your activity level and climate.

Moreover, incorporating regular physical activity into our routines dramatically impacts our skin. Exercise boosts circulation, ensuring that vital nutrients reach our skin cells, and enhances our overall well-being. This connection between physical health and skin appearance highlights the importance of adopting a lifestyle that prioritizes both.

The Importance of Tailored Skincare

Despite our best efforts, life inevitably poses challenges that can disrupt our routines and affect our skin. Stress, travel, and hormonal changes can lead to breakouts, dullness, or other skin concerns. During periods of hormonal fluctuations, such as puberty, menstruation, or menopause, it's essential to be adaptable with our skincare. Following a skincare regimen that is responsive to these changes can mitigate some of the adverse effects on our skin. This might include using gentle cleansers during hormonal surges to soothe acne-prone skin or hydrating masks to combat dryness during stressful times. Additionally, understanding when to invest in quality makeup products can help enhance our natural beauty, allowing us to feel confident even when our skin is less than perfect.

My philosophy on beauty extends far beyond surface-level treatments to embrace a holistic approach to skin health. This means:

- Selecting products specifically formulated for your unique skin type
- Experimenting thoughtfully to discover your skin's individual preferences and needs
- Prioritizing ingredients that support skin function rather than temporarily mask problems
- Avoiding harmful additives, fragrances, and irritants that can compromise skin health over time

This approach requires more initial effort than simply following trends but results in a personalized regimen that works with your skin's biology rather than fighting against it.

This chapter will offer insights into various skincare practices like cleansing, moisturizing, sun protection, and more—that can lead to healthier and radiant skin by taking specific actions to not only resist but potentially reverse skin aging.

Factors Contributing to Skin Aging

What are the primary factors contributing to skin aging? I would argue that there are five principal causes.

1) Nutrient Depletion

As we age, our ability to absorb vital nutrients diminishes. Furthermore, the nutritional quality of our food has significantly decreased. The food we consume today is significantly less nutritious than it was decades ago, when in fact, it should be more nutrient-dense given modern advances. Protein, iron, and vitamin C stand out among the essential nutrients. These three elements play crucial roles in maintaining skin health. Holistic health experts strongly advocate for the consumption of supplements and organic foods to counteract nutrient depletion effectively.

2) Collagen Degradation

Collagen comprises approximately 70% to 80% of our skin, providing it with a firm and taut appearance. Starting in our mid-twenties, we lose an estimated 1% of collagen yearly as we age. To mitigate this ongoing loss, it is essential to incorporate strategies into our daily routines that promote collagen production and preservation.

Interestingly, after menopause, the rate of collagen loss in women increases to approximately 2% per year. This accelerated decline elucidates why it is common to observe women in their 60's and 70's with notably thin skin.

Collagen is a significant protein in our bodies and a large complex molecule. Topical collagen creams are ineffective as they cannot penetrate the skin's barrier; thus, they do not increase collagen levels within the skin. It is a fallacy to believe that collagen creams can enhance the collagen content of your skin—they merely serve as moisturizers.

The debate surrounding collagen supplements is prominent: Do they actually contribute to enhancing the collagen in your skin? The evidence suggests that they can. Numerous studies have demonstrated that intake of hydrolyzed collagen peptide supplements can indeed improve skin collagen. Notably, a meta-analysis published in December 2021 in the International Journal of Dermatology reviewed a total of 1,125 participants aged between 20 and 70 years (95% women). In this meta-analysis, a grouped analysis of studies showed favorable results of hydrolyzed collagen supplementation compared with placebo in terms of skin hydration, elasticity, and wrinkles. Based on results, ingestion of hydrolyzed collagen for 90 days is effective in reducing skin aging, as it reduces wrinkles and improves skin elasticity and hydration (de Miranda, 2021).

Therefore, high-quality collagen supplements that contain hydrolyzed collagen peptides, which facilitate absorption and potential efficacy, should be incorporated into a daily regimen for skin wellness.

The Role of Protein Intake

Another critical inquiry is whether increasing dietary protein intake can improve collagen levels in the skin. The answer is probably 'YES'. Although there may not be extensive studies directly linking protein intake to skin quality, the logic stands that collagen itself is a form of protein. Consuming adequate amounts of protein is a fundamental consideration, especially to avoid sarcopenia—the age-related loss of muscle mass and strength. Therefore, adding a sufficient amount of high-quality protein and hydrolyzed collagen supplementation, in combination with strength and resistance training, presents a promising solution to aging.

The Role of Retinoids

Prioritizing products containing proven anti-aging ingredients like retinoids is widely regarded as the most effective anti-aging component. Retinoids, such as retinol, are paramount in building collagen in the skin. Retinoids are available in two primary forms: tretinoin, which requires a prescription, and retinol, available over the counter. For individuals with sensitive skin, starting with retinol is advisable, as it can effectively contribute to the stimulation of collagen synthesis.

From a holistic standpoint, increasing protein intake, supplementing with collagen, and utilizing retinoid products can combat collagen degradation, thereby significantly enhancing skin health.

3) Understanding Oxidation and Free Radicals

The third major cause of skin aging is oxidation or the presence of free radicals. Free radicals are harmful molecules produced as byproducts of our natural metabolic processes. They are essentially clusters of atoms that lack an electron, making them unstable and damaging to healthy cells and DNA.

A well-balanced diet and a healthy lifestyle enable the body to produce adequate natural antioxidants to counteract free radicals. However, an unhealthy lifestyle, such as smoking, pollution, or ultra-processed foods, can lead to oxidative stress, contributing to premature aging and cellular damage.

Prevention Strategies

So, how can we combat oxidation and free radicals? The first step is to consume plenty of antioxidants, which are abundant in fruits and vegetables.

Incorporating a variety of colors in our diet—green, red, orange, and yellow fruits and vegetables can significantly enhance our intake of antioxidants. The pigments in these fruits and vegetables are the sources of these vital antioxidants. This approach not only fortifies our body against free radical damage but also enhances overall health.

The Benefits of Vitamin C

From an inside-out perspective, Vitamin C offers numerous benefits for skin health. This essential nutrient can be ingested through various sources, including vitamin C-rich foods, particularly citrus fruits, or applied topically as a serum. I recommend utilizing both methods to maximize their effects on combating skin aging, oxidation, and free radicals.

4) Inflammation

Acute inflammation is the body's response to a cut or injury, initiating inflammation around the affected area. This inflammatory response is essential for facilitating healing and rejuvenation.

Certain treatments, such as laser and chemical peels, induce acute inflammation. This controlled inflammation plays a vital role in restoring skin health. In essence, acute inflammation is a positive bodily response that aids in healing, particularly following mild trauma to the skin.

On the other hand, chronic inflammation is our body's long-term response to injury and is harmful if left untreated. Chronic inflammation can result in constant damage to the skin, compounding the aging process. Sugar acts as the primary culprit for skin aging. Repeated sugar and insulin spikes subsequently lead to chronic inflammation, resulting in constant damage to the skin. The second significant way sugar contributes to premature skin aging is through glycation, which occurs when sugar molecules bind to collagen and elastin fibers in the skin (Danby, 2010). When sugar binds to collagen, it can cause the collagen fibers to kink. Kinked fibers lose their strength and resilience, resulting in sagging or loose skin—a common concern as we age.

High sugar consumption is a standard part of the Western diet. A staggering study revealed that sugary drinks, such as sodas, fruit juices, energy drinks, and other sweetened beverages that are often deceptively high in sugar content, account for approximately 40% of the caloric intake of many Americans (Witek, 2022).

So, what actionable steps can we take to reduce skin aging? Reducing sugar intake can significantly benefit our skin and overall health. One study estimates that a 20% reduction in sugar consumption could lead to substantial decreases in chronic inflammation and premature aging (Nguyen, 2015).

Additional manageable changes include substituting refined carbohydrates, such as white bread, white pasta, and white rice, with unrefined alternatives like whole grains. This simple dietary switch can effectively decrease sugar spikes, which will, in turn, help reduce chronic inflammation and slow the aging process.

5) The Impact of Cellular Waste Buildup

As our cells perform essential functions for our bodies, they also produce waste byproducts. This accumulation of waste can interfere with the intracellular processes in cells. When cells become overloaded with waste, their efficiency diminishes, leading to impaired functionality.

To combat this buildup of waste byproducts and promote youthful cellular function, our bodies engage in a process known as autophagy. Autophagy means "self-eating": an intrinsic recycling mechanism that allows the body to utilize old proteins and organelles for energy. This process facilitates the rejuvenation of the body, resulting in efficient cellular operations (Gomez-Virgiolio, 2022).

Autophagy declines with age; therefore, certain practices can be adopted to promote autophagy and enhance cellular cleansing, such as FASTING. Implementing intermittent fasting or other forms of caloric restriction can encourage your body to initiate autophagy more frequently, thus improving cellular health and functionality.

In today's fast-paced environment, we often find ourselves caught in a cycle of constant eating and snacking, frequently consuming meals immediately upon waking and just before bedtime. This habitual pattern does not allow our bodies the necessary rest period to recycle intracellular debris and waste products efficiently. Consequently, many anti-aging scientists advocate for intermittent fasting as a beneficial practice.

During the fasting period, consuming drinks with no calories, such as water, black coffee, or tea, is perfectly acceptable. It is important to avoid any caloric intake. The longer we allow our gut to rest, the more time our body has to engage in autophagy, potentially enhancing the restorative benefits.

Emphasizing Internal Wellness for External Beauty

Now, let's explore the interplay between skin health, aesthetics, and personal care practices to ensure our skin remains healthy between dermatologist visits. Simply put, our health reflects on our faces. However, I also recognize that life is unpredictable. Stress, travel, late nights, and hormonal fluctuations can occasionally leave us feeling less than our best. The pursuit of true beauty begins with prioritizing nutrition, hydration, and restorative sleep. My philosophy emphasizes the importance of skin health and achieving a natural radiance.

This chapter provides strategies and insights to inspire our journey toward optimal health from within. Every individual's path to wellness is unique. This awareness underscores the importance of having the right skincare regimen and utilizing skin-specific treatments, such as targeted lasers and tools, to maintain skin health.

Our skin, which comprises approximately 15% of our body weight, functions as a barometer of internal health. Visible issues such as redness or puffiness—often indicate underlying nutritional deficiencies or other systemic imbalances. Hydration levels, sleep quality, and diet significantly influence skin appearance and health.

While societal pressure about vanity exists, evolutionary biology imposes that attractiveness is associated with perceived health. Beautifying oneself can enhance self-esteem, confidence, and overall well-being.

Selecting the appropriate nutrition not only boosts energy levels and reduces disease risk but also enhances physical appearance.

In the following sections, I will outline a list of beauty superfoods that serve as essential building blocks for tissue support, development, and protection. Key dietary components such as fats and proteins are critical for healthy tissue formation, particularly collagen synthesis. Antioxidants, including vitamins A, C, and E, alongside zinc and selenium, protect against oxidative stress and environmental stressors. Foods promoting digestive health are paramount; efficient digestion and nutrient absorption are fundamental for sustaining vibrant skin, hair, nails, and overall wellness.

Optimal hydration is vital for cellular vitality. Sweating from exercise unclogs pores and enhances circulation, ensuring efficient nutrient delivery to all body cells. Sleep serves as a recovery period for cellular repair and detoxification; thus, balancing these key factors is essential.

The foundation of a beauty-enhancing diet comprises fresh fruits and vegetables, omega-3-rich healthy fats, and lean proteins.

Vitamin C, Antioxidants, and Phytonutrients

Citrus and Tropical Fruits: Fruits such as lemons, limes, grapefruit, oranges, mangoes, guavas, and papayas are rich in vitamin C, a potent antioxidant that shields cells from free radicals while facilitating collagen formation.

Colorful Plant-Based Foods: A vibrant array of colorful fruits and vegetables is rich in antioxidants, which not only provide diverse nutrients but also protect against cellular aging and inflammation.

Rich reds, deep purples, vibrant greens, and sunny yellows signify nutrient-dense options.

Blueberries, blackberries, and raspberries are abundant in fiber and antioxidants. For added flavor, consider sprinkling them with cinnamon.

Healthy Fats

Avocados are a nutrient-dense fruit. They are abundant in healthy fats, fiber, phytonutrients, antioxidants, and protein (around 6g), promoting skin health and overall vitality.

Eggs (Healthy fats + protein): Eggs promote collagen production and are a notable source of vitamin A, critical for cellular repair and rejuvenation. In particular, cooked egg yolks provide nearly the entire recommended dietary allowance (RDA) of biotin, a nutrient essential for healthy hair and nails.

Fish Oil (Omega-3 fatty acids): Wild Alaskan salmon and sardines improve cell integrity by supporting the protective fatty membranes around skin cells. Flaxseeds and chia seeds serve as effective omega-3 alternatives for those who abstain from fish.

Coconut Oil: Coconut oil enhances skin health and reduces inflammation. Incorporate it into your diet by adding it to smoothies, using it for cooking, or consuming a spoonful daily.

Protein

Eat enough protein from pasture-raised animals, eggs, wild-caught fish, and plant proteins (black beans or tofu for vegans and vegetarians). Consume an additional 30 grams of grass-fed collagen for connective tissue strength. In general, for easy and straightforward protein-requirement calculations, every individual should aim for at least 100 grams of protein per day for overall health and wellness.

Organic Whey Powder: A clean protein source, organic whey powder is a staple in my diet—just combine it with water/smoothies and a dash of cinnamon for a nutritious shake.

Nuts and Seeds

Pumpkin Seeds (zinc): Pumpkin seeds protect cellular membranes and are vital for collagen synthesis. They also aid in the prevention of acne-related breakouts.

Raw Almonds (Vitamin E): Essential for maintaining smooth and healthy skin and providing a substantial protein source.

Seeds: Flaxseeds, hemp seeds, and chia seeds are versatile additions to smoothies, oatmeal, or desserts, packed with proteins, fibers, and omega-3 fatty acids.

Fermented Foods (probiotics)

Products such as sauerkraut, kimchi, kombucha, yogurt, and kefir are rich in probiotics, enhancing digestive function and immunity. A balanced digestive system benefits skin, hair, and nail health and aids in weight management.

Hydration

Water: Essential for overall wellness, proper hydration enhances skin plumpness and vibrancy while aiding the detoxification process. Aim to drink water (oz.) approximately half of your body weight (lbs.).

Consumption of high-water-content foods such as cucumbers (96% water), tomatoes, watermelon, and radishes help maintain hydration.

Lemons: Lemon juice in water serves as a cleansing agent, promoting alkalinity and enhancing skin health.

Daily Ritual

Every morning: Kickstart your metabolism with a glass of warm lemon water mixed with cayenne pepper and a pinch of Celtic salt. This refreshing drink is a simple yet effective way to promote alkalinity. Additional superfoods like wheatgrass, dandelion leaves, chlorophyll, chlorella, and sprouts can be added for an energy boost.

Before meals: Apple cider vinegar helps lower blood sugar levels, improves insulin sensitivity, aids in reducing bloating, promotes clear skin, and enhances alkalinity. For consumption purposes, mix one teaspoon with a glass of water for a daily tonic before meals in order to slow the digestion of carbohydrates and lower blood sugar spikes after meals.

Harmful Ingredients to Avoid for Optimal Health and Skin Vitality

To achieve optimal health and radiant skin, it's essential to be mindful of the ingredients in the foods we consume daily.

1. Processed Food: Often contains preservatives, dyes, emulsifiers, and chemicals that are detrimental to health. These substances disrupt hormonal balance and deteriorate digestion, energy levels, and overall well-being.

2. Excess Salt: High sodium intake can lead to puffiness and swelling around the eyes. It also contributes to water retention throughout the body. Fast food, pre-packaged meals, and salty snacks are common culprits, but also pay attention to similar ingredients in canned soups, salad dressings, and breads.

3. Soda: They are high in sugar and artificial sweeteners, which provoke insulin spikes and also contribute to dehydration compromising skin health.

4. Sugar: Both refined sugar and high-fructose corn syrup disrupt blood sugar metabolism, energy fluctuation, and hormonal imbalance. Excess sugar intake is associated with various metabolic health diseases, like obesity, diabetes, and even cancer.

5. Additionally, excess sugar adversely affects gut microbiota, collagen and elastin degradation and accelerates skin aging.

6. White Flour: Commonly found in breads and baked goods, it triggers rapid blood sugar spikes, disrupting metabolic functions. Consider substituting with brown rice, quinoa, and almond flour as these are low glycemic index and more nutrient-dense options.

7. Alcohol: While enjoying a cocktail can be part of a social lifestyle, moderation is key.

Drinking too much alcohol damages the liver, disrupts blood sugar metabolism, and depletes vitamins, minerals, and fluids out of the body. It's advisable to limit your alcohol to 1-2 drinks/week or very occasionally. For individuals who suffer from a hangover, consuming plenty of hydrating fluids like coconut water (8 oz.), B-complex vitamins, foods rich in vitamin C, and bone broth with ginger is a little trick.

The Role of Supplements in Health and Vitality

Supplements address nutritional gaps that are often challenging to fill through food alone.

My baseline regimen includes fish oil, a probiotic, and vitamin D3.

For stress management, incorporate a B-complex vitamin that is essential in mood regulation and cognitive function.

Include magnesium, melatonin, and inositol, which help to calm the brain and nerves and facilitate relaxation for abundant beauty sleep.

Probiotics: A compromised gut barrier allows toxins to enter the bloodstream, leading to various skin conditions, including acne, psoriasis, dermatitis, and premature aging. Therefore, adding a potent probiotic might be beneficial. Be mindful that the probiotic contains at least 20 billion colony-forming units (CFUs), ideally those that require refrigeration to ensure live bacterial viability. It is advisable to alternate probiotic brands every 90 days to maintain a variety of bacterial strains.

The Importance of Sleep for Skin Health and Beauty

Insufficient sleep can manifest as dark circles under the eyes and dull skin. The National Sleep Foundation (NSF) recommends 7 to 9 hours of restorative sleep per night (Oyetakin-White, 2015). However, sleep quality, particularly the amount of rapid eye movement (REM) sleep, is crucial. Approximately 4 - 5 REM cycles alternating with non-REM stages are vital for waking up feeling refreshed, restored with muscle and tissue repair, and boosted immune function.

Comprehensive Skincare Routine

Our skin is not the same every day. It varies and therefore, maintaining a diligent skincare regimen is crucial for optimizing skin health and minimizing the signs of aging.

Daily Skincare Routine

Cleansing: A cleanser's job is to remove dirt, makeup, and impurities so do thorough research to choose a preferred cleanser that suits the skin's need. A personal tip: to reduce any swelling and puffiness in the morning, I always splash cold water on my face before using my cleanser. In the evening, a double cleanse is preferred: the first one is to remove the makeup and impurities, and the second is with a gentle AHA or BHA cleanser.

Toning: Toners and tonics to soothe, hydrate, and reduce buildup are the second steps after cleansing. Avoid using alcohol-based toners and look for water-based formulas with ingredients such as aloe, lavender, and cucumber.

Serums: Serums are packed with plenty of skin-nourishing ingredients that are more potent than our moisturizer and act on the deeper layers, targeting our skincare needs such as acne, lifting, fine lines, and hydration. Layer the serums immediately after cleansing and toning but before applying moisturizers to make sure active ingredients are fully absorbed in the skin.

Moisturizer: Every woman should have a daytime and nighttime moisturizer/cream for hydrated, plump, and smooth skin. The nighttime creams tend to be thicker and heavier than daytime moisturizers to provide intensive hydration and anti-aging benefits.

Sunscreen: Too much sun exposure damages collagen, causing skin wrinkles. Never skip sun protection. Always apply sunscreen with an SPF of 50 or higher to shield skin from harmful UV rays. For optimal protection, use a mineral sunscreen containing zinc oxide or titanium dioxide after applying moisturizer for broad-spectrum protection from UVA as well as UVB radiations. Try to limit sun exposure between 10 AM and 4 PM to protect the skin from harsh UV rays that are known to cause skin cancer, particularly melanoma.

Exfoliants: No matter what type of skin we have, we need to exfoliate on a regular basis to reveal smoother and fresher skin to allow skincare ingredients to penetrate more effectively. For face, choose a gentle exfoliant and customize this practice 2 - 3 times per week in your skincare routine. For the body, an oil paired with brown sugar or sea salt is an excellent exfoliating practice as often as needed to keep the skin smooth and moisturized.

Dry Brushing: Incorporating dry brushing from periphery to center into your daily routine can improve circulation, exfoliate dead skin cells, promote lymphatic drainage, and facilitate toxin removal. This process takes only a few minutes and can yield significant benefits.

Potent Skincare Ingredients

Achieving healthy, radiant skin starts with the right ingredients. Potent skincare ingredients have the power to transform our complexion by addressing concerns such as aging, hydration, fine lines, dryness, and texture.

Although these may sound like very dermatological ingredients, I did not want to end this chapter without sharing these powerful skincare ingredients to help you navigate what really works for skin transformation. These ingredients are most frequently packed in serums.

1. Growth Factors and Peptides: These powerful ingredients play a pivotal role in skin repair and regeneration and are commonly found in anti-aging products. Regular application, ideally twice daily, promotes collagen and elastin synthesis, leading to a noticeable improvement in skin texture over time.

2. Hyaluronic Acid: When applied, hyaluronic acid provides immediate plumping benefits, softens fine lines, and makes skin appear visibly firmer due to its moisture-retention properties.

3. Hydroxy Acids: Alpha hydroxy acids (AHAs) and beta hydroxy acids (BHAs) are vital to facilitating cell turnover. They effectively slough off dead skin layers to reveal fresh, new skin beneath, thereby softening fine lines and unclogging pores.

4. Retinol: A proven anti-aging powerhouse, retinol boosts collagen and elastin production, diminishes hyperpigmentation, and accelerates cell turnover through exfoliation. Due to its sensitivity to sunlight, it is best used at night. Start by applying retinol every other night, using only a dime-sized amount, to allow your skin to acclimate. Pair it with

soothing creams containing growth factors, peptides, or vitamin B3 to hydrate and calm the skin.

5. Vitamin C: This potent antioxidant brightens the complexion, reduces inflammation, diminishes the appearance of fine lines and wrinkles, and protects the skin from free radical damage. When layered under sunscreen, vitamin C enhances photoprotection, counteracting sun damage. Choose for serums or concentrates housed in dark bottles with a pump to minimize exposure to air and light, which can degrade their efficacy.

6. Vitamin B3 (Niacinamide): Vitamin B3 is an excellent option for sensitive skin. Its anti-inflammatory and soothing properties address redness and discoloration while strengthening the skin's barrier function.

Skin Treatments/Skincare Innovations

Spa treatments have evolved beyond simple massages and products. Innovative technologies, such as LED therapy, microcurrents, peels, radio frequency, ultrasound-based lasers, and ablative lasers, are now used for transformative results.

1. LED Therapy: Different colored lights serve various purposes; for instance, amber light addresses wrinkles, while blue light targets acne. Light-emitting diode (LED) therapy is a painless, non-invasive treatment that requires no recovery time, distinguishing it from laser procedures.

Research indicates that cells exposed to red LED light regenerate 150 to 200 percent faster. This therapy expedites the healing process by enhancing cellular energy production through adenosine triphosphate (ATP).

Red light therapy can enhance skin appearance, resulting in a more youthful, smoother, and firmer complexion.

Amber light specifically helps diminish wrinkles and inhibit matrix metalloproteinases (MMPs), enzymes linked to the aging process, elasticity loss, and brown spots caused by sun exposure.

Blue LED light therapy is notable for its ability to eradicate acne-causing bacteria, specifically Propionibacterium acnes. While individual results may vary based on factors like health, diet, skin color, and lifestyle, significant improvements are commonly observed with a treatment series of six to eight sessions. The combination of blue light for bacterial elimination with red light for regeneration offers an effective synergistic effect.

2. Microcurrents: When utilized effectively, advanced devices powered by specific microcurrents, such as the Resculpter, can lift, firm, and contour the jawline and cheekbones while minimizing puffiness and dark circles around the eyes.

3. Peels: Go for mild to medium chemical peels as they yield impressive results without the extreme redness or discomfort often associated with higher concentrations. While mild stinging may occur during the treatment, it should generally be painless.

These peels typically utilize a combination of alpha hydroxy acids, beta hydroxy acids, and retinoic acid to reveal a new layer of skin and minimize wrinkles, acne, and discoloration. One of my favorite peels is Vitalize Peel from SkinMedica. Note that peels available at a spa or dermatologist's office are the most effective.

4. Radio Frequency: Radio frequency (RF) devices are effective for toning and tightening the skin, with results potentially lasting up to two years. These devices are typically used with a coupling gel or an emulsion to deliver RF waves beneath the skin's surface. Some advanced devices combine RF technology with microneedling, resulting in a more intensive treatment.

- Profound RF: The Profound RF treatment is a needle-based radio frequency option that stimulates the production of elastin, collagen, and hyaluronic acid. It is unique in its ability to promote the synthesis of all three, effectively lifting and contouring sagging jawlines while restoring volume.

    I favor combining RF microneedling with platelet-rich plasma (PRP) treatment or exosomes, both of which are rich in growth factors that rejuvenate skin cells. These RF treatments enhance collagen production, improve skin tightening, reduce localized fat, and diminish sunspots, which are often early indicators of aging.

5. Ablative laser (Fraxel): The Fraxel laser treatment rejuvenates skin cells by creating micro-injuries that

stimulate collagen production beneath the surface. This powerful treatment effectively targets fine lines, wrinkles, sun damage, and scarring and promotes overall skin renewal. Fraxel is a proven technology that can help reverse visible signs of aging and texture. The only downside is five to seven days of redness, puffiness, and peeling sunburn appearance downtime.

- (Baby Fraxel) Clear + Brilliant is a gentle fractional laser treatment designed to stimulate collagen production. This laser method applies energy to targeted fractions of the skin while preserving the surrounding untreated area and therefore, has a faster healing process than fully ablative lasers. It effectively improves skin texture and tone, enhances radiance, and reduces the appearance of pores for a clearer, healthier complexion without the downtime.

6. Cool Sculpting: This technology freezes and destroys the fat cells, ensuring 20 - 25% in fat thickness in each treatment. It might be beneficial to those who have stubborn spots of fat on their thigh, hip, waist, and chin that cannot be eliminated by diet or exercise. It is the most effective non-invasive fat reduction technique with no scarring or downtime when compared to liposuction.

Overall, these treatments offer a less invasive alternative to plastic surgery.

In conclusion, beauty is a multifaceted concept that intertwines health, well-being, and personal expression. By focusing on what we put into our bodies and how we care for our skin, we can foster a lasting sense of confidence and self-love. I hope that the insights shared in this chapter will inspire you to take actionable steps toward enhancing your skin health. Remember, every journey is unique, and embracing our own path is essential to becoming the best version of ourselves—from the inside out.

Key Things to Do

Consider following some of the routines below to improve both skin health and overall wellness:

1. Follow a consistent skincare routine using gentle cleansers, toners, moisturizers, and serums best suited to your skin type.

2. Take high-quality hydrolyzed collagen supplements to maintain skin elasticity and increase dietary protein intake to support collagen production.

3. Maintain a balanced diet, including a variety of colorful fruits and vegetables, healthy fats, and high-quality protein.

4. Avoid smoking, pollution, and processed foods that increase free radical damage.

5. Limit sugar intake to prevent glycation, replace refined carbohydrates with whole grains, and reduce consumption of sugary drinks, processed foods, and excessive salt.

6. Implement intermittent fasting to enhance cellular waste removal and renewal.

7. Stay hydrated by drinking water equal to half your body weight (in oz.) daily. Start the day with warm lemon water to promote alkalinity and detoxification.

8. Limit processed foods with preservatives, excess salt, and refined sugar. Avoid white flour and opt for whole grains for better metabolic balance. Consume alcohol in moderation to prevent dehydration and nutrient depletion.

9. Incorporate supplements such as fish oil, probiotics, and Vitamin D3.

10. Prioritize sleep and strive to get 7-9 hours of quality sleep per night, focusing on achieving 4-5 REM cycles for optimal skin and body restoration.

11. Exfoliate 2-3 times per week with gentle acids or scrubs.

12. Dry brush before showering to improve circulation and detoxification.

13. Use potent skincare ingredients, like growth factors, peptides, hyaluronic acid, vitamin C, retinol, and hydroxy acids (AHA/BHA).

14. Explore advanced skincare treatments for fine lines, texture, and radiance, including LED therapy, microcurrent devices, and chemical peels.

CHAPTER 10

Movement, Strength, And Fitness – Foundation for Vitality

Exercise is the most powerful tool for promoting health and combating the effects of aging by improving heart, lung, brain, bones, muscle health, and mood. Studies show that exercise may improve longevity by delaying the onset of various chronic diseases, preventing cognitive decline, reducing the risk of falls, and alleviating stress and anxiety (Ruegsegger, 2018).

In other words, getting fit, burning fat, building muscle, and improving your strength and endurance are non-negotiable. The sooner you begin and the longer you remain physically active, the better. But getting fit does not have to mean running a marathon or spending hours in the gym. Any kind of movement, including taking the stairs, gardening, or walking the dog, has physical and cognitive benefits when done regularly.

Benefits of Exercise

The benefits of exercise as part of a healthy lifestyle cannot be understated for our overall health and well-being.

Just some of the many benefits include:

- Enhancing the health of blood vessels and muscles, lowering the risk of hypertension, type 2 diabetes, and cardiovascular disease.

- Supporting mitochondria to produce energy, burn fat, and build lean muscle mass

- Boosting the immune system, decreasing the risk of cancer

- Improving gut health

- Fighting inflammation, reducing the risk of heart disease, type 2 diabetes, stroke, and cancer, as well as depression and other mental health issues

- Enhancing cognitive health, preventing the onset of Alzheimer's disease

- Improving mobility and balance, reducing the risk of falls, fractures, and related injuries

Exercise Is Even More Crucial as We Age

Research suggests that muscle strength is a key predictor of healthy aging rather than sheer muscle mass (Cawthorn, 2018). However, despite the research and information available about the benefits of strength training, including improved metabolism, heart health, bone health, cognition, and overall wellness, three in five US adults do not engage in any muscle-strengthening exercise (Bennie, 2018).

As we age and experience a decline in bodily functions, causing us to naturally become sedentary and our muscles to atrophy due to lack of use, exercise becomes even more essential.

When we lack regular exercise, our muscles become impaired because they do not undergo the essential process of contraction and relaxation. This muscle disuse causes excess carbohydrates, fats, and sugar to build up in the bloodstream, leading to the accumulation of advanced glycation end products (AGEs) and further resulting in inflammation and increased risk of chronic diseases, like the risk of high blood pressure, stroke, cardiovascular disease, type 2 diabetes, Alzheimer's, and dementia.

Inactivity or lack of regular exercise impacts our body in the following detrimental ways:

Metabolism

Excess carbohydrates and fats in the body can lead to weight gain and various health conditions. Muscles use carbohydrates and fats for contraction, hence clearing the excess and avoiding the build-up of sugar in the bloodstream, as excess sugar in the blood leads to chronic inflammation and deposition of fat around the waistline, increasing the risk of high cholesterol, cardiovascular disease, and stroke.

Bone and Muscle Health

According to the National Osteoporosis Foundation, osteoporosis results from the decline of bone density and strength, costing the healthcare system $19 billion annually (Harding, 2020). Sarcopenia, the loss of muscle mass and function, occurs simultaneously due to overall decreased bone density and strength (Rosenburg, 1997; Cruz-Jentoft et al., 2010), begins in the mid-30s to 40s, and further decreases at the rate of 2 - 4% per year after age 60 (Goodpaster et al., 2006; Delmonico et al., 2009). Our day-to-day choices of activity can make a positive impact on our bone and muscle health. For example, engaging in weight-bearing exercises and resistance training just 2 - 3 times per week can significantly improve bone and muscle strength and overall health.

Biological Age

As we age, the length of telomeres (as discussed in Chapter 3) becomes shorter. However, research conducted by Brigham-Young University suggests that adding aerobic exercise to our exercise regimen may help to lengthen our telomeres, hence decreasing our biological age (Tucker, 2017).

Heart Health

The heart, which is a muscle, is most efficient when exercised and trained, like any other muscle in our bodies. Strength training can reduce risk factors associated with heart disease and lower blood cholesterol levels (Schroeder, 2019).

Another benefit of resistance training is reduced levels of inflammation, particularly high-sensitivity C-reactive protein (hsCRP), which is closely associated with improvements in cardiovascular health as well as overall fat loss and well-being (Martins, 2010).

Mental Health

As we age, our cognitive abilities to learn, remember, and react can diminish. Exercise improves brain function and enhances cognition by releasing brain-derived neurotrophic factor (BDNF), a chemical that increases neurogenesis. A 2020 study reveals that exercising for 20 minutes increases the blood flow to the hippocampus (memory and cognitive performance) area of the brain, improving our cognitive skills (Meng, 2020).

It has been discovered that strength training has other cognitive benefits, including mood enhancement and depression relief. Several studies conclusively indicate that resistance and strength training improve not only cognitive performance but also the overall quality of life in older adults (Khodadad, 2023).

Variety of Exercise Techniques

The following is a list of exercises to help get you moving and help you to effectively build lean muscle mass, effectively burn fat, and positively impact your overall well-being.

Aerobic Training

Aerobic training, such as running, cycling, and swimming, improves the cardiovascular system by strengthening the heart muscles, increasing blood volume and oxygen demand, thereby improving oxygen utilization in the muscles.

High-Intensity Interval Training (HIIT)

High-Intensity Interval Training (HIIT), which consists of short bursts of intense work for between 15 seconds to 4 minutes, is one of the most efficient ways to improve your cardiovascular fitness. The goal of this type of training is to raise the heart rate and maximize the volume of oxygen the body uses during exercise.

Some examples of HIIT training include vigorous walking, running, jump rope, weightlifting, cycling, stair climbing, and swimming sprints. Each interval or burst should be followed by an active recovery period.

Resistance/Strength Training

Resistance training is an exercise technique that increases muscle strength by making our muscles work against a weight or force. Different forms of resistance training include:

- Free weights (i.e., barbells, dumbbells, or kettlebells)
- Weight machines (i.e., lateral pull-down station, leg press machine)
- Resistance bands
- Body weight (i.e., push-ups, pull-ups, squats)

The form of strength training is not as important as ensuring that we push our muscles hard enough that they can gradually adapt to heavier weights and greater resistance.

Ideally, we should alternate working one body part or muscle group during each workout session, allowing for adequate rest and muscle recovery.

Despite its cardiovascular health benefits, HIIT is not as effective as resistance training at building muscle strength, which the body naturally loses in the aging process. Hence, it is essential to incorporate both forms of exercise to improve overall strength and endurance.

How Much Exercise Is Necessary?

It is not necessary to become a master athlete but just simply engaging in any level of activity is better than none.

- Adults should engage in a minimum of 150 - 300 minutes per week of moderate-intensity or 75 - 150 minutes of vigorous-intensity physical activity per week.

- Additionally, strength training or resistance exercise at moderate or greater intensity should be performed using all major muscle groups on 2+ days per week.

Exercise Intensity

To determine our physical activity intensity, it is essential to calculate our maximum heart rate (MHR) during exercise. This can be done using the formula (220 - current age). For example, a 40-year-old's maximum heart rate would be 180 beats per minute (bpm).

So, where should our heart rate be?

- Moderate intensity: ideally, stay within 50 - 70% of MHR
- Vigorous intensity: ideally, stay within 70 - 85% of MHR

Understanding these parameters can help ensure that we are exercising at the appropriate intensity for our fitness goals.

Protein Considerations for Exercise

Building and maintaining muscle is not solely dependent on the duration or intensity of strength training; it also requires proper recovery. Providing sufficient protein is essential to fuel the recovery process, which is just as important as the workout itself.

Protein intake:

- More than 65 years of age should consume 1.2 g/kg per day to maintain proper muscle mass
- Malnourished or injured adults should aim for 1.2 - 1.5 g/kg body weight per day
- General athletes/endurance athletes and runners should get 1.2 - 1.4 g/kg per day
- Strength athletes need 1.6 - 2.2 g/kg per day to maintain muscle mass

Post-exercise refueling for optimal muscle recovery and growth (anabolic window or muscle protein synthesis window):

- Women need 30 - 40 grams of protein post-exercise within a 90-minute window
- Men need a minimum of 20 grams within 3 hours post-exercise

Three essential amino acids (EAA), leucine, isoleucine, and valine, are crucial for muscle growth after exercise. As the body cannot produce these amino acids on its own, it is important to obtain them through diet or supplementation, particularly post-exercise, to enhance muscle recovery and stimulate protein synthesis, supporting overall muscle development.

Key Things to Do

Research consistently highlights the benefits of enhancing our overall health and health span. Although there is no specific exercise regimen that fits everyone's needs, there are several guidelines for achieving optimal health through exercise.

1. Take at least 1 day off each week, preferably 2.

2. Alternate the muscle groups throughout the week; never train a particular muscle group on 2 consecutive days.

3. Do not strength train a muscle if it is still sore from a previous workout.

4. To consistently achieve the benefits of exercise, it is essential to practice structured routines and progressive challenge.

5. Work out at least 30 minutes and up to 60 minutes 5 times per week.

6. Engage in weightlifting, bodyweight exercises, or resistance training to build and maintain muscle strength.

7. HIIT workouts should be done at least once per week, or low-intensity cardio at least twice per week.

8. Monitor post-exercise protein consumption within the above-stated timelines.

9. Prioritize getting 7 - 9 hours of quality sleep each night, as it is essential for muscle recovery, hormonal regulation, and overall health.

10. Ensure adequate hydration and mineral intake (sodium, potassium, magnesium, and calcium) before, during, and after exercise. Replacing these electrolytes is important for muscle function, nerve signaling, and preventing cramping.

11. Prioritize post-exercise nutrition by consuming a balanced meal rich in protein to aid in muscle recovery and overall performance.

12. Try to implement techniques like steam saunas and red-light saunas that significantly enhance muscle recovery.

13. Don't forget stretching, which is a fun way to cool down and prevent soreness.

CONCLUSION

The Stronger Path Forward

Aging is inevitable. But how we age is a choice. *Age Stronger, Live Longer* has been our guide to understanding and taking charge of that choice.

Across these chapters, we've uncovered the real science of longevity. Not the myths or magic pills but the actionable truth. We've explored how inflammation and insulin resistance are the hidden saboteurs of aging and how addressing root causes, rather than merely managing symptoms, is key to preventing disease. We've mapped out the terrain of optimal metabolic health, hormone balance, gut integrity, strength, sleep, skin vitality, and the power of nutrient-dense food and targeted supplementation.

What we now have is a blueprint for living with clarity, energy, and strength, regardless of age.

This book isn't about perfection. It's about awareness, agency, and alignment. Awareness of what our body truly needs, agency to make empowered choices, and alignment between our daily actions and our long-term goals for health and vitality.

Whether we are 35 or 65, it's never too early (or too late) to shift the trajectory of aging.

So, here's the invitation:

We should be our own best experiment.

Measure. Track. Reflect. Adjust.

Prioritize sleep. Lift weights. Eat protein. Heal our gut. Manage stress.

Our journey to optimal health and aging stronger doesn't end here. It begins with the very next choice we make. We are not at the mercy of time; we are in partnership with it. And the more we honor that partnership, the longer and better we will live.

References

Chapter 1

Anisimov, VN. "Effect of Epitalon on biomarkers of aging, life span and spontaneous tumor incidence in female Swiss-derived SHR mice." Biogerontology, vol. 4, no. 4, 2003, pp. 193-202. PubMed, https://pubmed.ncbi.nlm.nih.gov/14501183/.

BMJ. Association of fried food consumption with all cause, cardiovascular, and cancer mortality: prospective cohort study. 2019. The BMJ, https://www.bmj.com/content/364/bmj.k5420.

Gilbert, SF. Developmental Biology. 6 ed., Sunderland, Sinauer Associates, 2000. National Institutes of Health, https://www.ncbi.nlm.nih.gov/books/NBK10041/.

Hickson LJ, Langhi Prata LGP, Bobart SA, Evans TK, Giorgadze N, Hashmi SK, Herrmann SM, Jensen MD, Jia Q, Jordan KL, Kellogg TA, Khosla S, Koerber DM, Lagnado AB, Lawson DK, LeBrasseur NK, Lerman LO, McDonald KM, McKenzie TJ, Passos JF, Pignolo RJ, Pirtskhalava T, Saadiq IM, Schaefer KK, Textor SC, Victorelli SG, Volkman TL, Xue A, Wentworth MA, Wissler Gerdes EO, Zhu Y, Tchkonia T, Kirkland JL. Senolytics decrease senescent cells in humans: Preliminary report from a clinical trial of Dasatinib plus Quercetin in individuals with diabetic kidney disease. EBioMedicine. 2019 Sep;47:446-456. doi: 10.1016/j.ebiom.2019.08.069. Epub 2019 Sep 18. Erratum in: EBioMedicine. 2020 Feb;52:102595. PMID: 31542391; PMCID: PMC6796530.

Huat, Tee Jong. "Metal Toxicity Links to Alzheimer's Disease and Neuroinflammation." Journal of Molecular Biology, vol. 431, no.

9, 2019, pp. 1843-1868. PubMed, https://pubmed.ncbi.nlm.nih.gov/30664867/.

Lithgow, Gordon. "A new look at vitamin D challenges the current view of its benefits." Buck Institute, 18 October 2016, https://www.buckinstitute.org/news/a-new-look-at-vitamin-d-challenges-the-current-view-of-its-benefits/. Accessed 3 October 2023.

McHugh D, Gil J. Senescence and aging: Causes, consequences, and therapeutic avenues. J Cell Biol. 2018 Jan 2;217(1):65-77. doi: 10.1083/jcb.201708092. Epub 2017 Nov 7. PMID: 29114066; PMCID: PMC5748990.

Mohammed, I., Hollenberg, M. D., Ding, H., & Triggle, C. R. (2021). A Critical Review of the Evidence That Metformin Is a Putative Anti-Aging Drug That Enhances Healthspan and Extends Lifespan. Frontiers in Endocrinology, 12, 718942. https://doi.org/10.3389/fendo.2021.718942

Morgan, K. K. (2022, November 7). The Link Between Cancer and Your Age. WebMD. Retrieved October 3, 2023, from https://www.webmd.com/cancer/cancer-incidence-age

National Human Genome Research Institute. "Lysosome." National Human Genome Research Institute, https://www.genome.gov/genetics-glossary/Lysosome. Accessed 3 October 2023.

Niccoli, T. (2012, September 11). Aging as a Risk Factor for Disease. Current Biology, 22(17), R741-R752. https://www.sciencedirect.com/science/article/pii/S0960982212008159

Olshansky, S Jay. "Differences in life expectancy due to race and educational differences are widening, and many may not catch up." Health Aff (Millwood), vol. 8, no. 31, 2012, pp. 1803-1813. National Institutes of Health, https://pubmed.ncbi.nlm.nih.gov/22869659/.

Raghupathi, W. (2018). An Empirical Study of Chronic Diseases in the United States: A Visual Analytics Approach to Public Health. International Journal of Environmental Research and Public Health, 15(3), 431. https://www.ncbi.nlm.nih.gov/pmc/articles/PMC5876976/

Rogers, Kara. "Mitochondrion | Definition, Function, Structure, & Facts." Britannica, 1 October 2023, https://www.britannica.com/science/mitochondrion. Accessed 3 October 2023.

Shammas MA. Telomeres, lifestyle, cancer, and aging. Curr Opin Clin Nutr Metab Care. 2011 Jan;14(1):28-34. Doi: 10.1097/MCO.0b013e32834121b1. PMID: 21102320; PMCID: PMC3370421.

Shay, JW. "Hayflick, his limit, and cellular ageing." Nat Rev Mol Cell Biol, vol. 1, no. 1, 2000, pp. 72-76. PubMed, https://pubmed.ncbi.nlm.nih.gov/11413492/.

Sunderland P, Alshammari L, Ambrose E, Torella D, Ellison-Hughes GM. Senolytics rejuvenate the reparative activity of human cardiomyocytes and endothelial cells. The Journal of Cardiovascular Aging. 2023; 3(2): 21. http://dx.doi.org/10.20517/jca.2023.07

Song, Seonghyeok. "Does Exercise Affect Telomere Length? A Systematic Review and Meta-Analysis of Randomized Controlled

Trials." Medicina (Kaunas), vol. 5, no. 58, 2022, p. 242. PubMed, https://www.ncbi.nlm.nih.gov/pmc/articles/PMC8879766/.

Tedone, Huang. "Telomere length and telomerase activity in T cells are biomarkers of high-performing centenarians." Aging Cell, vol. 18, no. 1, 2018, p. e12859. National Library of Medicine, https://www.ncbi.nlm.nih.gov/pmc/articles/PMC6351827/.

Uribarri J, Woodruff S, Goodman S, Cai W, Chen X, Pyzik R, Yong A, Striker GE, Vlassara H. Advanced glycation end products in foods and a practical guide to their reduction in the diet. J Am Diet Assoc. 2010 Jun;110(6):911-16.e12. Doi: 10.1016/j.jada.2010.03.018. PMID: 20497781; PMCID: PMC3704564.

Yu Y, Zhou L, Yang Y, Liu Y. Cycloastragenol: An exciting novel candidate for age-associated diseases. Exp Ther Med. 2018 Sep;16(3):2175-2182. doi: 10.3892/etm.2018.6501. Epub 2018 Jul 20. PMID: 30186456; PMCID: PMC6122403.

Chapter 2

Alabadi B, Civera M, De la Rosa A, Martinez-Hervas S, Gomez-Cabrera MC, Real JT. Low Muscle Mass Is Associated with Poorer Glycemic Control and Higher Oxidative Stress in Older Patients with Type 2 Diabetes. Nutrients. 2023 Jul 17;15(14):3167. doi: 10.3390/nu15143167. PMID: 37513585; PMCID: PMC10383462.

Alzheimer's Disease Facts and Figures. (2023). Retrieved from Alzheimer's Association: https://www.alz.org/alzheimers-dementia/facts-figures

Anand P, Kunnumakkara AB, Sundaram C, Harikumar KB, Tharakan ST, Lai OS, Sung B, Aggarwal BB. Cancer is a preventable disease that requires major lifestyle changes. Pharm Res. 2008 Sep;25(9):2097-116. doi: 10.1007/s11095-008-9661-9. Epub 2008 Jul 15. Erratum in: Pharm Res. 2008 Sep;25(9):2200. Kunnumakara, Ajaikumar B [corrected to Kunnumakkara, Ajaikumar B]. PMID: 18626751; PMCID: PMC2515569.

Ask the Doctors - What is the cause of death in Alzheimer's disease? (2018, July 5). Retrieved from UCLA Health: https://www.uclahealth.org/news/ask-the-doctors-what-is-the-cause-of-death-in-alzheimers-disease

Cardiovascular Diseases. (2021, June 11). Retrieved from World Health Organization: https://www.who.int/news-room/fact-sheets/detail/cardiovascular-diseases-(cvds)

Cheung, V., Yuen, V.M., Wong, G.T.C. and Choi, S.W. (2019), The effect of sleep deprivation and disruption on DNA damage and health of doctors. Anaesthesia, 74: 434-440. https://doi.org/10.1111/anae.14533

Dementia. (2023, March 15). Retrieved from World Health Organization: https://www.who.int/news-room/fact-sheets/detail/dementia

Il'yasova D, Fontana L, Bhapkar M, Pieper CF, Spasojevic I, Redman LM, Das SK, Huffman KM, Kraus WE; CALERIE Study Investigators. Effects of 2 years of caloric restriction on oxidative status assessed by urinary F2-isoprostanes: The CALERIE 2 randomized clinical trial. Aging Cell. 2018 Apr;17(2):e12719. doi: 10.1111/acel.12719. Epub 2018 Feb 9. PMID: 29424490; PMCID: PMC5847862.

Murtaugh, E. M. (2010). Walking - the first steps in cardiovascular disease prevention. Current Opinion in Cardiology, 490-496.

References

National Aging Institute, Alzheimer's Disease Genetics Fact Sheet. 01 March 2023. https://www.nia.nih.gov/health/alzheimers-disease-genetics-fact-sheet

Obesity and Overweight. (2021, June 9). Retrieved from World Health Organization: https://www.who.int/news-room/fact-sheets/detail/obesity-and-overweight

Piffner Morgan, MS, Holmer, Brady (2023, August 16) Healthy Aging & Longevity https://examine.com/categories/healthy-aging-longevity/

Piotr Dobrowolski, e. a. (2022). Metabolic Syndrome - a new definition and management guidelines. Archives of Medical Science, 1133-1156.

Robinson, Matthew M., Dasari, Surendra, Konopka, Adam R., Carter, Ricky, E., et al. Enhanced Protein Translation Underlies Improved Metabolic and Physical Adaptations to Different Exercise Training Modes in Young and Old Humans. Clinical and Translational Report, Volume 25, Issue 3. 2017 March 7.

Simioni C, Zauli G, Martelli AM, Vitale M, Sacchetti G, Gonelli A, Neri LM. Oxidative stress: role of physical exercise and antioxidant nutraceuticals in adulthood and aging. Oncotarget. 2018 Mar 30;9(24):17181-17198. doi: 10.18632/oncotarget.24729. PMID: 29682215; PMCID: PMC5908316.

Shalev D, Arbuckle MR. Metabolism and Memory: Obesity, Diabetes, and Dementia. Biol Psychiatry. 2017 Dec 1;82(11):e81-e83. doi: 10.1016/j.biopsych.2017.09.025. PMID: 29110819; PMCID: PMC5712841.

Tafton, Anne. (2023, May 25) Exploring the links between diet and cancer: https://news.mit.edu/2023/omer-yilmaz-exploring-links-between-diet-and-cancer-0525#:~:text=In%20a%202018%20study%2C%20his,could%20have%20a%20beneficial%20effect.

Tsao, C. E. (2023, January 25). Heart Disease & Stroke Statistics 2023 Update. Retrieved from American Heart Association: https://www.heart.org/en/about-us/heart-and-stroke-association-statistics

Wang, W. Z. (2020). Mitochondria dysfunction in the pathogenesis of Alzheimer's disease; recent advances. Molecular Neurodegeneration, 15-37.

Waziry, R., Ryan, C.P., Corcoran, D.L. et al. Effect of long-term caloric restriction on DNA methylation measures of biological aging in healthy adults from the CALERIE trial. Nat Aging 3, 248–257 (2023). https://doi.org/10.1038/s43587-022-00357-y

What Is Atherosclerosis? (2022, March 24). Retrieved from National Institutes of Health: https://www.nhlbi.nih.gov/health/atherosclerosis

World Obesity Day 2022 – Accelerating action to stop obesity https://www.who.int/news/item/04-03-2022-world-obesity-day-2022-accelerating-action-to-stop-obesity

Noncommunicable diseases https://www.who.int/news-room/fact-sheets/detail/noncommunicable-diseases

Causes of death: Overview. Geriatrics. (2024, January 4). https://geriatrics.stanford.edu/ethnomed/alaskan/health_risk_patterns/death_causes.html#:~:text=The%20major%20cause%20of

%20death,%2C%20cerebrovascular%20diseases%2C%20and%20pneumonia

Cancer statistics. National Cancer Institute. (n.d.). https://www.cancer.gov/about-cancer/understanding/statistics

Chapter 3

U.S. Department of Health and Human Services. (n.d.). Goal A: Better understand the biology of aging and its impact on the prevention, progression, and prognosis of disease and disability. National Institute on Aging. https://www.nia.nih.gov/about/aging-strategic-directions-research/goal-biology-impact

Dariush Mozaffarian, M. (2008, May 12). Metabolic syndrome and mortality in older adults. Archives of Internal Medicine. https://jamanetwork.com/journals/jamainternalmedicine/fullarticle/414200#:~:text=Results%20At%20baseline%20(mean%20age,%5D%2C%201.11%2D1.34).

Ferrucci L, Fabbri E. Inflammageing: chronic inflammation in ageing, cardiovascular disease, and frailty. Nat Rev Cardiol. 2018 Sep;15(9):505-522. doi: 10.1038/s41569-018-0064-2. PMID: 30065258; PMCID: PMC6146930.

Guo, J., Huang, X., Dou, L., et al. Aging and aging-related diseases: from molecular mechanisms to interventions and treatments. Sig Transduct Target Ther 7, 391 (2022). https://doi.org/10.1038/s41392-022-01251-0

Liguori I, Russo G, Curcio F, Bulli G, Aran L, Della-Morte D, Gargiulo G, Testa G, Cacciatore F, Bonaduce D, Abete P. Oxidative stress, aging, and diseases. Clin Interv Aging. 2018 Apr

26;13:757-772. Doi: 10.2147/CIA.S158513. PMID: 29731617; PMCID: PMC5927356.

Salminen, Antero & Kauppinen, Anu & Kaarniranta, Kai. (2013). Inflammaging Signaling in Health Span and Life Span Regulation: Next Generation Targets for Longevity. Inflammation, Advancing Age and Nutrition: Research and Clinical Interventions. 323-332. 10.1016/B978-0-12-397803-5.00027-7.

Warraich UE, Hussain F, Kayani HUR. Aging - Oxidative stress, antioxidants and computational modeling. Heliyon. 2020 May 31;6(5):e04107. doi: 10.1016/j.heliyon.2020.e04107. PMID: 32509998; PMCID: PMC7264715.

Chapter 4

Childs E, de Wit H. Regular exercise is associated with emotional resilience to acute stress in healthy adults. Front Physiol. 2014 May 1;5:161. Doi: 10.3389/fphys.2014.00161. PMID: 24822048; PMCID: PMC4013452.

Crinnion WJ. Environmental medicine, part one: the human burden of environmental toxins and their common health effects. Altern Med Rev. 2000 Feb;5(1):52-63. PMID: 10696119.

M.L. Brusseau, M. Ramirez-Andreotta, I.L. Pepper, J. Maximillian, Chapter 26 - Environmental Impacts on Human Health and Well-Being, Editor(s): Mark L. Brusseau, Ian L. Pepper, Charles P. Gerba, Environmental and Pollution Science (Third Edition), Academic Press, 2019, Pages 477-499, ISBN 9780128147191, https://doi.org/10.1016/B978-0-12-814719-1.00026-4.

Pu F, Chen W, Li C, Fu J, Gao W, Ma C, Cao X, Zhang L, Hao M, Zhou J, Huang R, Ma Y, Hu K, Liu Z. Heterogeneous associations of multiplexed environmental factors and multidimensional aging metrics. Nat Commun. 2024 Jun 10;15(1):4921. doi: 10.1038/s41467-024-49283-0. PMID: 38858361; PMCID: PMC11164970.

U.S. Department of Health and Human Services. (2024b, June 17). Making a healthier home. National Institutes of Health. https://newsinhealth.nih.gov/2016/12/making-healthier-home

Chapter 5

Al-Atif H. Collagen Supplements for Aging and Wrinkles: A Paradigm Shift in the Fields of Dermatology and Cosmetics. Dermatol Pract Concept. 2022 Jan 1;12(1):e2022018. Doi: 10.5826/dpc.1201a18. PMID: 35223163; PMCID: PMC8824545.

An SY, Lee MS, Jeon JY, Ha ES, Kim TH, Yoon JY, Ok CO, Lee HK, Hwang WS, Choe SJ, Han SJ, Kim HJ, Kim DJ, Lee KW. Beneficial effects of fresh and fermented kimchi in prediabetic individuals. Ann Nutr Metab. 2013;63(1-2):111-9. doi: 10.1159/000353583. Epub 2013 Aug 17. PMID: 23969321.

Center for Disease Control, Micronutrient Facts, March 2024 https://www.cdc.gov/nutrition/features/micronutrient-facts.html?CDC_AAref_Val=https://www.cdc.gov/nutrition/micronutrient-malnutrition/micronutrients/index.html

Filippo Ravalli, Xavier Vela Parada, Francisco Ujueta, Rachel Pinotti, Kevin J. Anstrom, Gervasio A. Lamas and Ana Navas-Acien

Originally published Mar 2022
https://doi.org/10.1161/JAHA.121.024648 Journal of the American Heart Association. 2022;11:e024648

Jozefczak M, Remans T, Vangronsveld J, Cuypers A. Glutathione is a key player in metal-induced oxidative stress defenses. Int J Mol Sci. 2012;13(3):3145-3175. doi: 10.3390/ijms13033145. Epub 2012 Mar 7. PMID: 22489146; PMCID: PMC3317707.

Morelli MB, Santulli G, Gambardella J. Calcium supplements: Good for the bone, bad for the heart? A systematic updated appraisal. Atherosclerosis. 2020 Mar;296:68-73. doi: 10.1016/j.atherosclerosis.2020.01.008. Epub 2020 Jan 29. PMID: 32033778; PMCID: PMC7276095.

Rafati-Rahimzadeh M, Rafati-Rahimzadeh M, Kazemi S, Moghadamnia AA. Current approaches of the management of mercury poisoning: need of the hour. Daru. 2014 Jun 2;22(1):46. doi: 10.1186/2008-2231-22-46. PMID: 24888360; PMCID: PMC4055906.

Soemarie YB, Milanda T, Barliana MI. Fermented Foods as Probiotics: A Review. J Adv Pharm Technol Res. 2021 Oct-Dec;12(4):335-339. doi: 10.4103/japtr.japtr_116_21. Epub 2021 Oct 20. PMID: 34820306; PMCID: PMC8588917.

U.S. National Academies of Sciences, Engineering, and Medicine, Report Sets Dietary Intake Levels for Water, Salt, and Potassium To Maintain Health and Reduce Chronic Disease Risk, 2004 February 11.
https://www.nationalacademies.org/news/2004/02/report-sets-dietary-intake-levels-for-water-salt-and-potassium-to-maintain-health-and-reduce-chronic-disease-risk

Chapter 6

Andrea Di Francesco et al., A time to fast. Science 362,770-775(2018).DOI:10.1126/science.aau2095

Centers for Disease Control and Prevention. (2022b, June 3). Defining adult overweight & obesity. Centers for Disease Control and Prevention. https://www.cdc.gov/obesity/basics/adult-defining.html#:~:text=Adult%20Body%20Mass%20Index&text=If%20your%20BMI%20is%20less,falls%20within%20the%20obesity%20range.

Chazelas E, Pierre F, Druesne-Pecollo N, Esseddik Y, Szabo de Edelenyi F, Agaesse C, De Sa A, Lutchia R, Gigandet S, Srour B, Debras C, Huybrechts I, Julia C, Kesse-Guyot E, Allès B, Galan P, Hercberg S, Deschasaux-Tanguy M, Touvier M. Nitrites and nitrates from food additives and natural sources and cancer risk: results from the NutriNet-Santé cohort. Int J Epidemiol. 2022 Aug 10;51(4):1106-1119. doi: 10.1093/ije/dyac046. PMID: 35303088; PMCID: PMC9365633.

Czarnecka K, Pilarz A, Rogut A, Maj P, Szymańska J, Olejnik Ł, Szymański P. Aspartame-True or False? Narrative Review of Safety Analysis of General Use in Products. Nutrients. 2021 Jun 7;13(6):1957. doi: 10.3390/nu13061957. PMID: 34200310; PMCID: PMC8227014.

Flanagan EW, Most J, Mey JT, Redman LM. Calorie Restriction and Aging in Humans. Annu Rev Nutr. 2020 Sep 23;40:105-133. Doi: 10.1146/annurev-nutr-122319-034601. Epub 2020 Jun 19. PMID: 32559388; PMCID: PMC9042193.

Jeong SH, Kang D, Lim MW, Kang CS, Sung HJ. Risk assessment of growth hormones and antimicrobial residues in meat. Toxicol

Res. 2010 Dec;26(4):301-13. Doi: 10.5487/TR.2010.26.4.301. PMID: 24278538; PMCID: PMC3834504.

Lee DH, Giovannucci EL. Body composition and mortality in the general population: A review of epidemiologic studies. Exp Biol Med (Maywood). 2018 Dec;243(17-18):1275-1285. doi: 10.1177/1535370218818161. Epub 2018 Dec 11. PMID: 30537867; PMCID: PMC6348595.

Liu S, Zeng M, Wan W, Huang M, Li X, Xie Z, Wang S, Cai Y. The Health-Promoting Effects and the Mechanism of Intermittent Fasting. J Diabetes Res. 2023 Mar 3;2023:4038546. Doi: 10.1155/2023/4038546. PMID: 36911497; PMCID: PMC10005873.

Mariotti F, Gardner CD. Dietary Protein and Amino Acids in Vegetarian Diets-A Review. Nutrients. 2019 Nov 4;11(11):2661. doi: 10.3390/nu11112661. PMID: 31690027; PMCID: PMC6893534.

McDonald RB, Ramsey JJ. Honoring Clive McCay and 75 years of calorie restriction research. J Nutr. 2010 Jul;140(7):1205-10. doi: 10.3945/jn.110.122804. Epub 2010 May 19. PMID: 20484554; PMCID: PMC2884327.

Nationalacademies.org. (n.d.). https://www.nationalacademies.org/news/2004/02/report-sets-dietary-intake-levels-for-water-salt-and-potassium-to-maintain-health-and-reduce-chronic-disease-risk

Niaz K, Zaplatic E, Spoor J. Extensive use of monosodium glutamate: A threat to public health? EXCLI J. 2018 Mar 19;17:273-278. doi: 10.17179/excli2018-1092. PMID: 29743864; PMCID: PMC5938543.

References

Olney JW. Excitotoxins in foods. Neurotoxicology. 1994 Fall;15(3):535-44. PMID: 7854587.

Papadopoulou SK. Sarcopenia: A Contemporary Health Problem among Older Adult Populations. Nutrients. 2020 May 1;12(5):1293. doi: 10.3390/nu12051293. PMID: 32370051; PMCID: PMC7282252.

Pifferi, F., Terrien, J., Marchal, J., et al. Caloric restriction increases lifespan but affects brain integrity in grey mouse lemur primates. Commun Biol 1, 30 (2018). https://doi.org/10.1038/s42003-018-0024-8

Pipoyan D, Stepanyan S, Stepanyan S, Beglaryan M, Costantini L, Molinari R, Merendino N. The Effect of Trans Fatty Acids on Human Health: Regulation and Consumption Patterns. Foods. 2021 Oct 14;10(10):2452. doi: 10.3390/foods10102452. PMID: 34681504; PMCID: PMC8535577.

Potera C. The artificial food dye blues. Environ Health Perspect. 2010 Oct;118(10):A428. doi: 10.1289/ehp.118-a428. PMID: 20884387; PMCID: PMC2957945.

Selsby JT, Judge AR, Yimlamai T, Leeuwenburgh C, Dodd SL. Life long calorie restriction increases heat shock proteins and proteasome activity in soleus muscles of Fisher 344 rats. Exp Gerontol. 2005 Jan-Feb;40(1-2):37-42. doi: 10.1016/j.exger.2004.08.012. PMID: 15664730.

Song DK, Kim YW. Beneficial effects of intermittent fasting: a narrative review. J Yeungnam Med Sci. 2023 Jan;40(1):4-11. doi: 10.12701/jyms.2022.00010. Epub 2022 Apr 4. PMID: 35368155; PMCID: PMC9946909.

Suzuki M, Wilcox BJ, Wilcox CD. Implications from and for food cultures for cardiovascular disease: longevity. Asia Pac J Clin Nutr. 2001;10(2):165-71. doi: 10.1111/j.1440-6047.2001.00219.x. PMID: 11710359.

U.S. Department of Health and Human Services. (n.d.). Autoimmune diseases. National Institute of Environmental Health Sciences. https://www.niehs.nih.gov/health/topics/conditions/autoimmune

Watson R. EU says growth hormones pose health risk. BMJ. 1999 May 29;318(7196):1442. doi: 10.1136/bmj.318.7196.1442a. PMID: 10346767; PMCID: PMC1115840.

Chapter 7

Brzecka A, Leszek J, Ashraf GM, Ejma M, Ávila-Rodriguez MF, Yarla NS, Tarasov VV, Chubarev VN, Samsonova AN, Barreto GE, Aliev G. Sleep Disorders Associated With Alzheimer's Disease: A Perspective. Front Neurosci. 2018 May 31;12:330. doi: 10.3389/fnins.2018.00330. PMID: 29904334; PMCID: PMC5990625.

Cappuccio FP, D'Elia L, Strazzullo P, Miller MA. Sleep duration and all-cause mortality: a systematic review and meta-analysis of prospective studies. Sleep. 2010 May;33(5):585-92. doi: 10.1093/sleep/33.5.585. PMID: 20469800; PMCID: PMC2864873.

Cooper CB, Neufeld EV, Dolezal BA, Martin JL. Sleep deprivation and obesity in adults: a brief narrative review. BMJ Open Sport Exerc Med. 2018 Oct 4;4(1):e000392. doi:

10.1136/bmjsem-2018-000392. PMID: 30364557; PMCID: PMC6196958.

Easton, J. (2016, February 29). Sleep loss boosts hunger and unhealthy food choices. UChicago Medicine. https://www.uchicagomedicine.org/forefront/news/sleep-loss-boosts-hunger-and-unhealthy-food-choices

Garbarino S, Lanteri P, Bragazzi NL, Magnavita N, Scoditti E. Role of sleep deprivation in immune-related disease risk and outcomes. Commun Biol. 2021 Nov 18;4(1):1304. Doi: 10.1038/s42003-021-02825-4. PMID: 34795404; PMCID: PMC8602722.

Garner, D. (2019b). Eat sleep burn.

Goldman, S. (2023, January 26). Lack of sleep and Alzheimer's risk. Comprehensive Sleep Care. https://comprehensivesleepcare.com/2022/04/18/lack-of-sleep-and-alzheimers-risk/#:~:text=Research%20is%20ongoing%2C%20but%20so,dementia%20risk%20in%20the%20future.

Greer SM, Goldstein AN, Walker MP. The impact of sleep deprivation on food desire in the human brain. Nat Commun. 2013;4:2259. doi: 10.1038/ncomms3259. PMID: 23922121; PMCID: PMC3763921.

Hafner, Marco, Martin Stepanek, Jirka Taylor, Wendy M. Troxel, and Christian Van Stolk, Why sleep matters — the economic costs of insufficient sleep: A cross-country comparative analysis. Santa Monica, CA: RAND Corporation, 2016. https://www.rand.org/pubs/research_reports/RR1791.html.

Blue Light has a dark side. Harvard Health. (2020, July 7). https://www.health.harvard.edu/staying-healthy/blue-light-has-a-dark-side

Kline CE. The bidirectional relationship between exercise and sleep: Implications for exercise adherence and sleep improvement. Am J Lifestyle Med. 2014 Nov-Dec;8(6):375-379. doi: 10.1177/1559827614544437. PMID: 25729341; PMCID: PMC4341978.

Liu Y, Wheaton AG, Chapman DP, Cunningham TJ, Lu H, Croft JB. Prevalence of Healthy Sleep Duration among Adults — United States, 2014. MMWR Morb Mortal Wkly Rep 2016;65:137–141. DOI: http://dx.doi.org/10.15585/mmwr.mm6506a1external icon

Mark Michaud (2023, June 13). Study that shows how brain cleans itself while we sleep honored by AAAS. URMC Newsroom. https://www.urmc.rochester.edu/news/story/study-that-shows-how-brain-cleans-itself-while-we-sleep-honored-by-aaas

Obesity and sleep. Sleep Foundation. (2023, December 22). https://www.sleepfoundation.org/physical-health/obesity-and-sleep

Staff, L. S. (2013b, May 30). Sleep is important to weight loss, research suggests. LiveScience. https://www.livescience.com/36652-sleep-weight-loss-advice.html#:~:text=They%20all%20cut%20their%20daily,tissue%2C%20and%20instead%20lost%20muscle.

Dr. Matthew Walker on sleep for enhancing learning, creativity, immunity, and Glymphatic System. FoundMyFitness. (n.d.).

2019 https://www.foundmyfitness.com/episodes/matthew-walker

Westwood AJ, Beiser A, Jain N, Himali JJ, DeCarli C, Auerbach SH, Pase MP, Seshadri S. Prolonged sleep duration as a marker of early neurodegeneration predicting incident dementia. Neurology. 2017 Mar 21;88(12):1172-1179. doi: 10.1212/WNL.0000000000003732. Epub 2017 Feb 22. PMID: 28228567; PMCID: PMC5373785.

Chapter 8

Blood sugar test - blood. Mount Sinai Health System. (n.d.). https://www.mountsinai.org/health-library/tests/blood-sugar-test-blood

By, & Knudsen, M. (2024, April 21). The 48 blood biomarkers InsideTracker measures. The InsideGuide. https://blog.insidetracker.com/blood-biomarker-testing

Centers for Disease Control and Prevention. (2022, September 8). Heart disease and stroke. Centers for Disease Control and Prevention. https://www.cdc.gov/chronicdisease/resources/publications/factsheets/heart-disease-stroke.htm#:~:text=The%20Nation's%20Risk%20Factors%20and,unhealthy%20diet%2C%20and%20physical%20inactivity.

Schaefer EJ, Santos RD, Asztalos BF. Marked HDL deficiency and premature coronary heart disease. Curr Opin Lipidol. 2010 Aug;21(4):289-97. doi: 10.1097/MOL.0b013e32833c1ef6. PMID: 20616715; PMCID: PMC6942922.

Sikaris K. The correlation of hemoglobin A1c to blood glucose. J Diabetes Sci Technol. 2009 May 1;3(3):429-38. doi:

10.1177/193229680900300305. PMID: 20144279; PMCID: PMC2769865.

U.S. Department of Health and Human Services. (n.d.). Office of dietary supplements - zinc. NIH Office of Dietary Supplements. 2022 https://ods.od.nih.gov/factsheets/Zinc-HealthProfessional/

U.S. Department of Health and Human Services. (n.d.-a). Office of dietary supplements - vitamin D. NIH Office of Dietary Supplements. 2023 https://ods.od.nih.gov/factsheets/VitaminD-HealthProfessional/

Vijay, A., Valdes, A.M. Role of the gut microbiome in chronic diseases: a narrative review. Eur J Clin Nutr 76, 489–501 (2022). https://doi.org/10.1038/s41430-021-00991-6

Chapter 9

Danby F. W. (2010). Nutrition and aging skin: sugar and glycation. Clinics in dermatology, 28(4), 409–411. https://doi.org/10.1016/j.clindermatol.2010.03.018

de Miranda RB, Weimer P, Rossi RC. Effects of hydrolyzed collagen supplementation on skin aging: a systematic review and meta-analysis. Int J Dermatol. 2021 Dec;60(12):1449-1461. doi: 10.1111/ijd.15518. Epub 2021 Mar 20. PMID: 33742704.

Gómez-Virgilio, L., Silva-Lucero, M. D., Flores-Morelos, D. S., Gallardo-Nieto, J., Lopez-Toledo, G., Abarca-Fernandez, A. M., Zacapala-Gómez, A. E., Luna-Muñoz, J., Montiel-Sosa, F., Soto-Rojas, L. O., Pacheco-Herrero, M., & Cardenas-Aguayo, M. D. (2022). Autophagy: A Key Regulator of Homeostasis and Disease: An Overview of Molecular Mechanisms and Modulators. Cells, 11(15), 2262. https://doi.org/10.3390/cells11152262

Nguyen, H. P., & Katta, R. (2015). Sugar Sag: Glycation and the Role of Diet in Aging Skin. Skin therapy letter, 20(6), 1–5.

Oyetakin-White, P., Suggs, A., Koo, B., Matsui, M. S., Yarosh, D., Cooper, K. D., & Baron, E. D. (2015). Does poor sleep quality affect skin ageing? Clinical and experimental dermatology, 40(1), 17–22. https://doi.org/10.1111/ced.12455

Witek K, Wydra K, Filip M. A High-Sugar Diet Consumption, Metabolism and Health Impacts with a Focus on the Development of Substance Use Disorder: A Narrative Review. Nutrients. 2022 Jul 18;14(14):2940. doi: 10.3390/nu14142940. PMID: 35889898; PMCID: PMC9323357.

Chapter 10

Bennie JA, Lee DC, Khan A, Wiesner GH, Bauman AE, Stamatakis E, Biddle SJH. Muscle-Strengthening Exercise Among 397,423 U.S. Adults: Prevalence, Correlates, and Associations With Health Conditions. Am J Prev Med. 2018 Dec;55(6):864-874. doi: 10.1016/j.amepre.2018.07.022. Epub 2018 Oct 24. PMID: 30458949.

Cawthon PM, Travison TG, Manini TM, Patel S, Pencina KM, Fielding RA, Magaziner JM, Newman AB, Brown T, Kiel DP, Cummings SR, Shardell M, Guralnik JM, Woodhouse LJ, Pahor M, Binder E, D'Agostino RB, Quian-Li X, Orwoll E, Landi F, Orwig D, Schaap L, Latham NK, Hirani V, Kwok T, Pereira SL, Rooks D, Kashiwa M, Torres-Gonzalez M, Menetski JP, Correa-De-Araujo R, Bhasin S. Establishing the Link Between Lean Mass and Grip Strength Cut Points With Mobility Disability and Other Health Outcomes: Proceedings of the Sarcopenia Definition and Outcomes Consortium Conference. J Gerontol A Biol Sci Med

Sci. 2020 Jun 18;75(7):1317-1323. Doi: 10.1093/gerona/glz081. PMID: 30869772; PMCID: PMC7447857.

Cruz-Jentoft AJ, Baeyens JP, Bauer JM, Boirie Y, Cederholm T, Landi F, Martin FC, Michel JP, Rolland Y, Schneider SM, Topinková E, Vandewoude M, Zamboni M; European Working Group on Sarcopenia in Older People. Sarcopenia: European consensus on definition and diagnosis: Report of the European Working Group on Sarcopenia in Older People. Age Ageing. 2010 Jul;39(4):412-23. doi: 10.1093/ageing/afq034. Epub 2010 Apr 13. PMID: 20392703; PMCID: PMC2886201.

Delmonico MJ, Harris TB, Visser M, Park SW, Conroy MB, Velasquez-Mieyer P, Boudreau R, Manini TM, Nevitt M, Newman AB, Goodpaster BH; Health, Aging, and Body. Longitudinal study of muscle strength, quality, and adipose tissue infiltration. Am J Clin Nutr. 2009 Dec;90(6):1579-85. doi: 10.3945/ajcn.2009.28047. Epub 2009 Oct 28. PMID: 19864405; PMCID: PMC2777469.

Goodpaster BH, Park SW, Harris TB, Kritchevsky SB, Nevitt M, Schwartz AV, Simonsick EM, Tylavsky FA, Visser M, Newman AB. The loss of skeletal muscle strength, mass, and quality in older adults: the health, aging and body composition study. J Gerontol A Biol Sci Med Sci. 2006 Oct;61(10):1059-64. Doi: 10.1093/gerona/61.10.1059. PMID: 17077199.

Harding AT, Weeks BK, Lambert C, Watson SL, Weis LJ, Beck BR. Effects of supervised high-intensity resistance and impact training or machine-based isometric training on regional bone geometry and strength in middle-aged and older men with low bone mass: The LIFTMOR-M semi-randomized controlled trial. Bone. 2020 Jul;136:115362. doi: 10.1016/j.bone.2020.115362. Epub 2020 Apr 11. PMID: 32289518.

References

Khodadad Kashi S, Mirzazadeh ZS, Saatchian V. A Systematic Review and Meta-Analysis of Resistance Training on Quality of Life, Depression, Muscle Strength, and Functional Exercise Capacity in Older Adults Aged 60 Years or More. Biol Res Nurs. 2023 Jan;25(1):88-106. Doi: 10.1177/10998004221120945. Epub 2022 Aug 13. PMID: 35968662.

Martins RA, Neves AP, Coelho-Silva MJ, Veríssimo MT, Teixeira AM. The effect of aerobic versus strength-based training on high-sensitivity C-reactive protein in older adults. Eur J Appl Physiol. 2010 Sep;110(1):161-9. doi: 10.1007/s00421-010-1488-5. Epub 2010 May 1. PMID: 20437055.

Meng Q, Lin MS, Tzeng IS. Relationship Between Exercise and Alzheimer's Disease: A Narrative Literature Review. Front Neurosci. 2020 Mar 26;14:131. doi: 10.3389/fnins.2020.00131. PMID: 32273835; PMCID: PMC7113559.

Ruegsegger GN, Booth FW. Health Benefits of Exercise. Cold Spring Harb Perspect Med. 2018 Jul 2;8(7):a029694. Doi: 10.1101/cshperspect.a029694. PMID: 28507196; PMCID: PMC6027933.

Rosenberg IH. Sarcopenia: origins and clinical relevance. J Nutr. 1997 May;127(5 Suppl):990S-991S. doi: 10.1093/jn/127.5.990S. PMID: 9164280.

Schroeder EC, Franke WD, Sharp RL, Lee DC. Comparative effectiveness of aerobic, resistance, and combined training on cardiovascular disease risk factors: A randomized controlled trial. PLoS One. 2019 Jan 7;14(1):e0210292. Doi: 10.1371/journal.pone.0210292. PMID: 30615666; PMCID: PMC6322789.

Tucker, Larry A. Physical activity and telomere length in U.S. men and women: An NHANES investigation. Preventative Medicine, Volume 100, pgs. 145-151. https://doi.org/10.1016/j.ypmed.2017.04.027.

www.ingramcontent.com/pod-product-compliance
Lightning Source LLC
Chambersburg PA
CBHW020543030426
42337CB00013B/954